THE LONG ROAD BACK TO BOSTON: RUNNING
MARATHONS WITH LEUKEMIA

Printed in the United States of America
First Printing, 2019
Print ISBN: 978-1-54395-850-8
eBook ISBN: 978-1-54395-851-5

BookBaby
7905 N. Crescent Blvd
Pennsauken, NJ 08110

I dedicate this book to all the women who have passed through my life. I am who and where I am today thanks to them.

You will learn who they are in this book.

THE **LONG ROAD BACK** TO **BOSTON**:

Running Marathons With Leukemia

Phillip Fields, Ph.D.

TABLE OF CONTENTS

SECTION I:
LEUKEMIA VS PASSION

SECTION II:
RUNNING MARATHONS WITH LEUKEMIA

INTRODUCTION

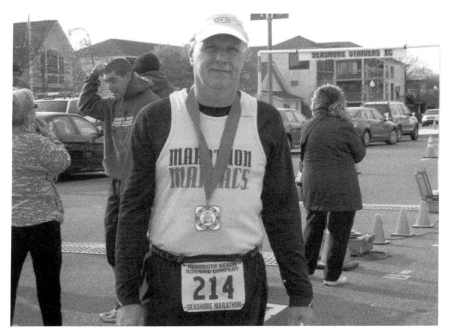

Rehoboth Seashore Marathon, DE (2010)

Dream as if you'll live forever.
Live as if you'll die today.
James Dean[1]

I am not sure who is responsible for this quote: "Bad news travels in threes." Well, my "threes" came in 2008 while sitting in an oncologist's office at The University of Texas MD Anderson Cancer Center in Houston, Texas. First, the oncologist confirmed

1

that I had leukemia and would soon require chemotherapy. Then, he informed me that the average life expectancy with my cell markers was five to seven years.

What made this a three-fer? He advised me to stop running for fear of rupturing my spleen or causing a hemorrhage. Following this advice—or rather, this directive—would prove easier said than done. Far easier. For me, not being able to run was the worst of the three pieces of bad news. You see, running is my passion, my "why". Now, more than ever, it is why (and how) I have been able to manage the diagnosis of leukemia, life expectancy numbers, chemotherapy, and everything else tossed my way.

I am not an elite runner. I am not even a good runner, but I am decent enough to have qualified for the Boston Marathon; however, you will not find any race trophies adorning my shelves.

Even though I am not among the privileged when it comes to running ability, I enjoy lacing up my running shoes each day and savor my time pounding the pavement. Not being able to do so disrupts my psyche and makes me depressed and grumpy. In other words, I am not fun to be around when I cannot run.

My dad once told me, "When doctors tell me that I can no longer smoke my pipe, they can cut my head off and throw it in the coffin with my dead body." Being only eight years old when I heard that, his logic seemed rather extreme.

I never assumed I would live forever, but prior to 2008, I had never given much thought to dying. Now, I understand what Dad was saying. We are all going to die, so we may as well die doing what we love. According to the poet Frank O'Hara, "We fight for what we love, not are."[2]

What I did next may seem foolhardy, but it was what I needed more than medicine, chemotherapy, or doctors. After briefly following the oncologist's advice, I decided to run again. More than that, actually, I would take my running to a new level. In February 2009, I began a journey to run a marathon in every state plus Washington, D.C. by the end of December 2012. (That would be fifty-one marathons in forty-seven months.) I would challenge my limits and that of this leukemia.

More than one person commented, "Are you crazy? Why try to finish by the end of December 2012? What is the rush?"

These people could not appreciate the fact that the sand was rapidly escaping from my (metaphorical) hourglass. My first symptoms appeared in December 2006, and Dr. Butler diagnosed me with leukemia in November 2007. When I made this goal in 2009, I was already two-to-three years into my life expectancy of five-to-seven years. Besides, without setting a time limit, my goal was nothing more than a passing thought. It was something that I had not yet considered to be worthy of completing.

Consequently, I would use leukemia to my advantage as it attempted to hasten the sand escaping from my hourglass of life. This would become my excuse to travel. I would visit all those places in our country that had long been on my list to see. In other words, I, not leukemia, would do the dictating, at least for now. I stopped racing the clock and began racing leukemia to the finish line of my goal. I felt like I was now racing against the angel of death.

If you are reading this book, you probably fall into one of a few categories. If you are a runner, you will be able to relate to many of my adventures. Maybe you are a cancer patient or a family member of one. You, too, will be able to connect with many of the stories in this book. In fact, there is something for everyone.

After all, this is a memoir. In these pages, you will find me writing about love, family, childhood stories, friendship, eating, drinking, war, history, and poetry. There is humor, tragedy, travel advice, adventure, animals, and insects, too. Of course, there are also stories about running.

As you read each chapter, see if you can discover where the title of each chapter originated. I liken this to looking for the sewing needle on one of the pages in the magazine *Country*. The quote at the beginning of each chapter represents the premise of that chapter. The photos are those I took during my travels. A "Chapter-Related Memory" at the end of various chapters is a recollection that surfaced during the writing of that chapter.

This book has two sections. Section I describes my initial diagnosis with leukemia. Woven into this section is how I developed a passion for running marathons, especially the Boston Marathon. Section II describes my attempt to accomplish my goal of running a marathon in every state with leukemia.

My aspirations for this book are numerous: One of them is to offer reasons to believe in God. Others are to provide a tribute to my mom; to recognize those individuals who helped me confront the harsh reality of cancer; and to remember the people in my life's journey who helped shape my belief system and my character. These people are partially responsible for my successes. They pointed me in the right direction and led by example. However, even though they prepared, aided, and nurtured me, the rest was up to me. I took those experiences and shaped them into my future. Consequently, I alone am responsible for my failures.

There are people who leave footprints in the sand, and some even on the moon. More important are those who have left their footprints in my heart. Their footprints, like those of the dinosaurs that archeologists have found fossilized deep in the earth, will remain with me forever.

I hope to inspire you, the reader, to never give up on living and never stop doing what you enjoy in life. Bob Hanson, race director for the Prairie Fire Marathon (Wichita, Kansas) and special friend, began his e-mail race updates with "Challenge your limits; don't limit your challenges."

I am optimistic that my journey will serve as a useful road map for yours.

SECTION I:

LEUKEMIA VS PASSION

CHAPTER 1

The Diagnosis

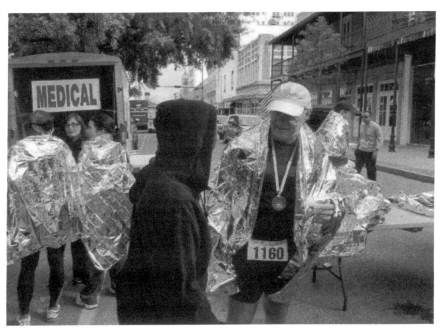

First Light Marathon, Mobile (2007)

The oldest and strongest emotion of mankind is fear.
And the oldest and strongest kind of fear is fear of the unknown.

H. P. Lovecraft[3]

It was 7 a.m. when I pulled off I-10 and into a gas station in Biloxi, Mississippi. My mission: Purchase a cup of coffee and a bag of unshelled sunflower seeds. The act of cracking the shells with my teeth and eating the seeds helps me stay awake on long drives. The purpose of the coffee was to provide an empty container for the sunflower shells; I forgot to bring one.

The date was January 28, 2008, and I was only one hour out of Mobile, Alabama. I was traveling west, toward The University of Texas MD Anderson Cancer Center in Houston, Texas. With another seven hours of driving time, the sunflower seeds were going to be indispensable for keeping me awake. Otherwise, a ditch might have ended up as the receptacle for the sunflower shells—and my truck.

The route, at least, was familiar. I had made this drive in April yearly since 1992. The purpose was to join family and friends for my Uncle Jim's birthday celebration. Since 1992, The University of Texas School of Public Health has sponsored a four-day event in his honor called the Annual James H. Steele Lecture. Dignitaries from around the world attend; Uncle Jim had sponsored, trained, or mentored most of them.

In April 2013, we celebrated his 100th birthday. The caterer decorated the cake with a plastic number 100, as we doubted the fire marshal would allow the burning of 100 candles.

There would not be a 101st birthday. Yet, despite Uncle Jim's passing, the Annual James H. Steele Lecture continues. Remembering this makes me stop and think, *What will my legacy be? How will people remember me?*

I will be pleased if people remember me as someone who cared and shared, who thought of others before himself, and who created more laughter than tears.

On those April trips, the bluebonnets were always in full bloom. They lined each side of the Texas highway with a radiant bouquet of cobalt blue. After the drab brown coloring of the winter months, the yearly renewal of springtime foliage rejuvenated my spirits. Spring marks not only a rebirth of plants, grasses, and trees but also a time of renewal for me.

As a professor at The University of South Alabama College of Medicine in Mobile, Alabama, I use this season to assess my achievements at work and in my personal life. When the first blooms of dogwood trees and azalea bushes make their appearance, I know it is time for self-evaluation: Have I been too self-centered, and do I need to do a better job of reaching out to others? I ask myself how I can improve, and then I try my best to do so.

Like the dogwood trees and azalea bushes in Mobile, the bluebonnet is symbolic of the arrival of spring in Texas.

There is a legend about how the Comanche were gifted this beautiful flower. A little girl, "She Who Is Alone", lived with the Comanche. Her heart was as big as Texas, and her spirit was as beautiful as the bluebonnet.

According to the legend, the land was suffering from a terrible drought. No matter what the rain dancers attempted, there was no relief. The shaman told the people that the Great Spirit believed they had become too selfish. For the rains to return, the Comanche had to offer a burnt sacrifice of their most valued possessions. The people gave offerings of knives, tomahawks, bows and arrows, and blankets. Nothing appeased the Great Spirit.

She Who Is Alone knew exactly what the Great Spirit expected: the doll she loved so dearly. That night, she went to the fire and offered her doll as a sacrifice, burning it and then scattering its ashes to the four corners of the earth. When the tribe arose the next morning, bluebonnets covered the hillsides, a sign of forgiveness from the Great Spirit. As they offered their thanks, the rains came and healed the earth.

This legend speaks to our need to take stock of what truly is most important in our lives, what we can live without and, more importantly, what we cannot. Soon, I would have to make that choice.

On those spring journeys to Houston, God also rewarded me with magnificent sunsets of pastel oranges, purples, and pinks. Sunsets are more resplendent when viewed in person. Only then can we truly comprehend their splendor. My mom was an artist, as well as a nurse, and she once told me, "Never waste a sunrise or sunset. Like lithographs of a painting by a great artist, they are numbered."

Now, it was January 28, 2008, when I pulled out from the gas station onto I-10 in Biloxi, Mississippi, with a cup of coffee and a bag of unshelled sunflower seeds, and nothing was in bloom. Everything was brown except for evergreen trees that sparsely dotted the landscape. Moreover, there would be no stunning sunset that evening. The sky was gray with gathering rain clouds.

This was a depressing trip, to be honest. It was a trip that I took alone, which turned out to be a bad idea.

To understand fully why I made this journey to Houston, I need to take you back to December 2006. I had just run the First Light Marathon in Mobile, Alabama, in order to log a long training run. I was preparing for the New Orleans Mardi Gras Marathon in February 2007, where I would attempt to qualify for the 2008 Boston Marathon.

My first Boston Marathon was in 1996, the 100th anniversary of the race. I was forty-eight years old. It was then that I set a goal to qualify every eight years for the Boston Marathon.

My preference was not to run the Boston Marathon too often; I wanted it to remain special amongst all my races. True to my goal, eight years later I qualified for the 2004 Boston Marathon. After that one, my inner voice beseeched me, *Do not wait another eight years*. This was an inner voice in the Christian tradition— the voice for which I searched and to which I listened. Having heard it, I set my sights on the 2008 Boston Marathon.

There is an old Yiddish proverb, "Man plans and God laughs." I do not think, though, that God really laughs at us, but the saying drives home the point that things can go wrong—and go wrong, they did.

Several weeks after the First Light Marathon, I could not complete a three-mile run without walking. It was as if someone had sucked all of the oxygen out of my body. When things did not improve, I canceled my trip to New Orleans and registered for a later marathon in Athens, Ohio (April 2007). I speculated, *Surely, things will return to normal in a couple of months*.

No such luck. My running deteriorated even further, and I canceled my trip to Athens, Ohio. My goal of returning to Boston was at risk, and I sought medical help. Because the onset of my problem had been so rapid, I made an appointment in May 2007 with a cardiologist, Dr. Chad Alford, one of my former students.

He ordered a nuclear stress test with a Doppler echocardio-gram. The results ruled out a heart problem, and he referred me to other specialists. During the next five months, I underwent pulmonary tests, and upper and lower GI tests. Being unable to discern a health-related reason for my running difficulty, one of the specialists said, "You appear to be a poster child for the physically fit. It is possible that your age is catching up with your running." I believe he thought I was exaggerating my problem. He even told me, "After all, you are still capable of running three miles each day. There are only a small percentage of men in Mobile your age doing that."

He did not fully appreciate my concern; I was accustomed to running a marathon in three hours and thirty minutes (3:30). I considered myself a couch potato when running only three miles. What this doctor simply did not comprehend was that runners know their bodies better than anyone else does. We know whether we are getting slower due to aging versus a medical issue. I was only fifty-nine years old and had effortlessly run a recent marathon. My problem was not due to aging.

With an absence of any medical reason for my fatigue, I simply assumed (or hoped) I would return to normal. Yet, things did not get better, and I continued to struggle with my running.

In October 2007, I went in for my yearly physical with Dr. Sforzini. Except for the fatigue I was experiencing, there was no particular problem. As usual, the physician performed the standard physical exam and drew blood in order to check my lipid, thyroid and liver profile, and my prostate-specific antigen level. Bingo! Nine months after running the First Light Marathon, the doctor detected something abnormal. My blood test indicated an elevated white blood cell count. The normal range is between 4,500 and 10,000 white blood cells per microliter; mine was 25,000.

Amazingly, that was the first blood test any doctor had requested during all those previous physical exams. I guess specialists can easily become so wrapped up in their areas of expertise that they sometimes overlook the obvious, the elementary.

Dr. Sforzini began palpating behind my ears, around my neck, in my armpits, and in my groin. He calmly informed me, "All your major lymph nodes are enlarged."

As he was jotting down notes, I inquired, "Is this why I am struggling with my running?"

Of course, I knew the answer was yes. After all, having enlarged lymph nodes throughout your body is never a good sign. I was hesitant to ask but did so anyway, "So what do you think is wrong?"

"Phillip, there are three things that will cause an elevated white blood cell count and enlarged lymph nodes. I do not want to overreact and alarm you, so we are going to rule out the possibilities one at a time."

In his attempt not to terrify me, he only told me about one pathology at a time. I did not express my frustration, but I thought to myself, *I'm expected to wait patiently a week for results from the first test. Then, if that test is negative, you will tell me what the next test will be. That is supposed to keep me from worrying?*

The first potential condition was mononucleosis and only required a blood test. I reasoned that my problem was not the "kissing disease." I had been divorced for almost two and a half years and had all but forgotten what a kiss was. Yet, as I anxiously awaited the results of that first test, I was fearful, not of the mononucleosis test results, but of what was behind door number two.

When the test for mononucleosis came back negative, I asked, "Okay, Doc, what is the second possibility?"

Without the slightest pause, he said, "HIV."

I was briefly stunned. That certainly was not on my radar of potential issues. I responded, "Well, that explains your probing questions about my sexual habits in our previous meeting. You are the first doctor who has asked me those sorts of questions. I suppose that should have tipped me off to what was next."

This, too, required a blood test and another week of waiting for the results. Because of my lifestyle, I should not have worried. However, those three letters, *HIV*, were enough to make a seven-day wait for results a fretful time. During that week, I recalled scenes from the movie *Philadelphia*. I even began looking in the mirror to see if there were any dark splotches on my body—Kaposi sarcoma (a type of cancer). Sleep did not come easily that week.

This test was negative as well, and with the lifting of my anxiety, I was feeling rather secure.

"So, Doc, why didn't you save that one for last? What can be worse than HIV?"

With a solemn look, he quietly responded, "You most likely have leukemia or lymphoma. I need to set up an appointment for you with an oncologist to confirm my diagnosis."

Wow! I thought, *That is getting right to the point.* Then again, that had been my first choice. I rather knew what he was going to say. Yet, at the same time, I was hoping he would not say it.

It is a jolt when a doctor says you have cancer. It is almost as bad as receiving a phone call late in the evening telling you that someone in your family has died. It is like having someone strike you in the solar plexus. The air empties from your lungs, and you can only stare awkwardly into space as you attempt to adjust to what has just happened.

Then Dr. Sforzini's last comment registered: "An oncologist needs to confirm my diagnosis." I began to feel more positive and thought, *I still have hope. Until there is confirmation, maybe things are not so bad.* I began, unknowingly, erecting a barrier against knowing.

As I left the doctor's office, I had one final thought: *I still think HIV would have been worse, and I would have saved that test for last.*

CHAPTER 2
The Confirmation

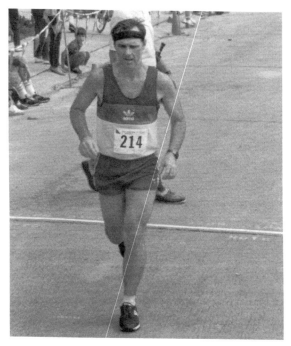

Mardi Gras Marathon, New Orleans (1985)

Bad news isn't wine. It doesn't improve with age.
Colin Powell[4]

As the lonely road to Houston stretched out before me, on that January 28, 2008 drive, the rather rude voice of a woman interrupted my daydreaming. "Recalculating!" I had been focusing so much on my musings that I failed to hear my GPS's announcement to stay left. I missed a lane change that would have taken me over the bridge and out of Baton Rouge, Louisiana. Thanks to my GPS, I was able to navigate through some not-so-appealing areas of the city and get back on track. I pondered, *How did I ever get by in the past with just a road map?* Back on I-10, I was still five hours away from Houston.

Between Baton Rouge and Lafayette, Louisiana, a stretch of I-10 is a bridge. This is an eighteen-mile double-span bridge over the Atchafalaya River and its adjoining lakes and uninhabitable swampland. The Atchafalaya Basin is the largest wetland in the United States and easily the most scenic portion of my trip.

Atchafalaya is a word from the Choctaw Indians and means "long river." As I drove (and drove, and drove), I concurred with their naming of this waterway. All that water had prompted a pit stop. My bladder was ready to pop, and there was nowhere to pull off on that long bridge for a private outing. I drove for what seemed like an eternity, sitting rigidly in the seat and doing Kegel exercises to keep from wetting my pants. My bladder was attempting to react as if I had my fingers submerged in ice water.

Thankfully, just as the situation seemed beyond my control, I reached the end of the bridge and then the exit for Lake Charles, Louisiana. The Kegel exercises had worked, and I did not have to change my pants. Departing Lake Charles, I was still three hours away from Houston.

• • •

Let me get back to the reason for the trip. Dr. Sforzini had made an appointment for me to see an oncologist at the Mitchell Cancer Institute in Mobile, Alabama. My appointment was in one week

(November 2007). I continued running, as running was the one thing that kept me sane through all of this.

I went to that oncologist's meeting with high expectations. After agonizing for nearly ten months, I would now learn about my condition. I would be able to put all this worrying behind me and move on with my life. When someone tells me I may have leukemia or lymphoma, I want clarification. If the doctors are going to open Pandora's Box, I do not want to wait weeks to learn the particulars. At least, that was what I initially thought I wanted. As I would learn, there are times when you do not necessarily want to know. I had yet to contemplate that this might be only the first step toward larger issues. Beyond simply getting back to my normal routine and running, I had not thought this all the way through.

As it turned out, nothing would be normal again.

The oncologist at the Mitchell Cancer Institute was Dr. Thomas Butler, and he seemed a bit young to have a full understanding of blood cancers. Then again, I generally question the knowledge of anyone younger than I am. Nevertheless, I thought, *He seems pleasant enough, and I will wait to pass final judgment.*

First, the nurse collected a blood sample. In fact, from that point on, every doctor's visit would begin with the collection of a blood sample. There was always another needle.

Dr. Butler then palpated my lymph nodes and said, "Your lymph nodes are enlarged."

This came as no surprise, since I had been checking them myself on a daily basis since my visit with Dr. Sforzini. The proper palpation of lymph nodes is something I teach in medical anatomy.

Next, I lay on my back. With one of his hands pressing against my anterior abdominal wall below my ribs, he instructed, "Take a deep breath and hold it. Let it out." This was done on the right side where my liver is, and then on the left side where my spleen is located. "Your liver and spleen feel normal. They aren't enlarged." That was reassuring—two fewer issues I had to deal with.

Then Dr. Butler said he would schedule me for a bone marrow biopsy. You guessed it, in one week.

The earth was no longer spinning. The world's clock had stopped. It had now been more than a month since I had learned about my abnormal white blood cell count and enlarged lymph nodes. I still had no solution from any doctor for those issues. I had no solution for my deteriorating running.

Things never move fast enough when you are waiting for your scheduled clinical examination or when you are waiting for the results of one. Especially, when you know that the news is going to be bad. My mood suffered from the delays.

I was unaware that the waiting game was only beginning. Unfortunately, this was not a bottle of wine; I could not simply remove the cork and smell it to discern immediately just how far gone the wine was.

In my impatience during the week of waiting to have the biopsy done, I read numerous medical articles about leukemia and lymphoma. I learned about the various cell markers from my scheduled bone marrow biopsy that the pathologist would be evaluating. While Dr. Butler performed the biopsy, I inquired about these markers. I immediately realized that it would have been better had I inquired before he started. He had just shoved the trocar into my hipbone, and at my question, he stopped. My inquiry prompted him to call the pathologist. It was important to know which markers the pathologist would evaluate and how much marrow fluid he required for the tests.

At the time, with that large instrument protruding from my hip, I found this rather strange. I thought to myself in frustration, *Shouldn't the oncologist be telling the pathologist which markers to evaluate?* That was my justification later for requesting a second opinion. I eventually became secure with Dr. Butler's decisions, but at that time, I felt uneasy.

The pathologist obviously had answered Dr. Butler's question, since he finished collecting the bone marrow and removed the huge trocar from my hipbone, much to my relief. I would learn the results in one week.

(Just as a side note, if you ever require a bone marrow biopsy, accept all drugs that the doctor offers you. I did not. Why? People told me, "It won't be that bad." This was only the first of three bone marrow biopsies that I would eventually endure, and I never accepted the drugs I was offered. I kept telling myself, *I am tough, and this cannot get worse.* However, I realized that I am not tough, and it did get worse.

After another week of sleepless nights, I met with Dr. Butler to discuss the results of the biopsy. I sat in a chair in the examining room waiting for Dr. Butler to enter. I felt like a defendant in a courtroom, waiting for the jury to enter after their deliberation. I had no clue what having leukemia meant to my life. Would I be able to run again, or would having it be a death sentence? For me, not being able to run is a death sentence.

When Dr. Butler entered the room with my chart in his hand, I could tell by his body language that the news was not good. At that point, not wanting to hear the inevitable, I believe my brain went into a protective mode. As Dr. Butler began to speak, I felt like my body was present but my mind had gone elsewhere. His voice sounded distant and fuzzy in my ears. It was as if someone had turned the volume down on my radio; his words were incoherent, muffled, and difficult to decipher even if I had been trying. He was saying something about numbers and names of cell markers that were abnormal. I vaguely remember hearing something about a cell marker that the pathologist had trouble getting information about—there was not enough marrow volume or the technician messed up the assay. I did not comprehend fully the reason. It did not matter; it was too much information to attempt to digest.

Then Dr. Butler's voice became loud, as if someone had turned up the volume of my radio. "The bottom line is your B-lymphocytes are abnormal. You have chronic lymphocytic leukemia."

After that proclamation, the doctor's voice sounded again as though it was coming from a distant room. I am sure he was telling me something important, but my mind had again exited the premises. (Neurologists refer to this as "psychogenic syndrome." The brain receives an electrical shock when you receive dreadful news. It then retreats to a more comfortable zone.)

While my brain retreated, I attempted to comprehend what I had just heard. *I have leukemia, a blood cancer. Is it curable? What do I do now? Do I continue working? More importantly, what does this mean regarding my running?*

That last thought snapped me back to reality, back to his office, and back to our conversation.

I blurted out, "Can I continue to run?"

"We'll discuss that later," he answered. "First. . . ."

That add-on word sent my mind reeling again, and I had no idea what he had said. I was too busy formulating my own game plan.

I rejoined the conversation. "I would like to get a second opinion at MD Anderson Cancer Center. Can you set up an appointment?"

Many people are reluctant to ask their doctor to make an appointment for a second opinion. They are afraid it is insulting to the doctor. Yet, many years ago, I attended a seminar by one of the top neurologists in the country who said, "If your doctor will not make an appointment for you for a second opinion, fire him."

Dr. Butler graciously made an appointment for me with Dr. Keating at the MD Anderson Cancer Center in Houston, Texas. I felt confident as I thought, *This is one of the premier cancer centers for the treatment of leukemia and lymphoma. Surely, they will get me back to my normal running routine.*

Of course, this was only another false sense of security. I kept telling myself that I wanted to be sure of the diagnosis. However, looking back, I believe I was attempting to delay facing the reality that I had cancer. I was simply putting off the inevitable: the time when I would have to admit that I was no longer normal—or that my time was more limited than I had believed.

Before leaving for Houston, I had one further test conducted: a full body CT scan (**Chapter Related Memory: The CT Cocktail**. The story is at the end of the chapter).

The CT scan indicated enlarged lymph nodes throughout my body cavities. Yet, I found at least one positive thing about the result: I did not have tumors in any of my body organs. I took that as a victory: a glass half-full instead of a glass half–empty.

• • •

When I reached Beaumont, Texas, Houston was only two hours away; my destination was in sight. I could not actually see the Houston skyline, but it felt close.

That long drive reminded me of waiting for results and the next doctor's appointment—time seemed to stand still. Of course, with nothing to do but drive, I had plenty of time for deliberating about my situation. I did not have sufficient information to come to grips with the life-threatening aspect of leukemia. Had I paid attention to Dr. Butler and asked more questions, I would have known what to expect. I kept telling myself, *There will be plenty of time for this once I know more about my condition. This is no big deal.*

I was unaware that I was attempting to quarantine myself behind a self-imposed wall of denial because I did not want to know. Instead, I only managed to develop a terrible anxiety, with an ominous cloud of speculation constantly overhead. Now, my wall was disintegrating. My wait was ending. The sense of security that I had carefully constructed by repudiating my diagnosis was about to disappear. Soon, this visit would force me into knowing. Soon, I would have an answer to a recurring question, "Will I feel better knowing or not knowing?"

Chapter Related Memory: The CT Cocktail

Before leaving for Houston, I had one further test conducted: a full body CT scan.

After signing in at the radiology desk at the University of South Alabama Medical Center in Mobile, Alabama, I took a seat in the waiting room. A technician appeared with a 1,500-ml graduated container that he had filled to the top with a pink liquid. A straw was included along with verbal instructions: "This solution will coat the inside of your GI tract and provide the contrast needed for the scan. Drink it slowly over the next hour." It was a foul-tasting drink and I required every bit of an hour to empty the container.

As I was attempting to finish my drink, another patient signed in, sat down, and received a similar drink. Before the technician had time to provide the patient with instructions, the man took the container from the technician and knocked down that drink as if he were competing in a beer-guzzling contest. It took him less than ten seconds to empty the container.

The technician had the most incredulous look on his face as he stated, "You are not supposed to drink it all at once. It needs time to coat the inside of your GI tract. Shortly, I will bring you another, but drink it slowly this time."

As I watched this interaction, I thought, *No way! They would have to reschedule me because I would not be able to drink any more of that liquid today.* Not this guy. He responded, "Oh. Okay." He sounded like he looked forward to drinking more.

Later, when the technician returned with another 1,500-ml container of pink liquid for the man, I held up my container and proudly announced, "All gone."

About fifteen minutes later, the technician escorted me to the CT lab. As I left the waiting area, I turned to the man and said, "Good luck with that drink." We both laughed.

CHAPTER 3
Loss of Identity

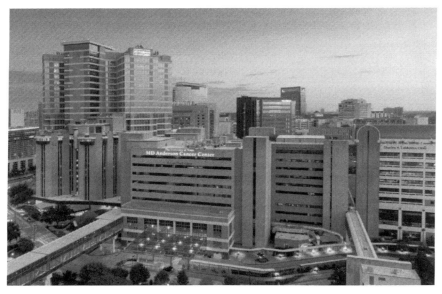

MD Anderson Cancer Center, Houston (2007)

Forgiveness is not an occasional act;
it's a permanent attitude.

James Van Praagh[5]

Most of my aimless thoughts during that trip focused on running. After all, that is what this illness threatened—my running. Now, more than any other time, I needed running to help me think about something other than leukemia.

The situation was harshly ironic. Doctors recommended that I not participate in high-impact sports—such as running. This could cause hemorrhaging that is associated with leukemia. Moreover, leukemia was compromising my immune system, and running might worsen the condition. Yet, at fifty-nine years old, I was not mentally prepared to give up my passion. I was not ready to give up running marathons.

• • •

I am not sure why I have this love affair with marathons. Maybe I enjoy them because of their uniqueness. Unlike anything else I do, a marathon allows me to push myself beyond what I consider my limit of physical endurance. There is a real sense of accomplishment in crossing the finish line and knowing that I have given my best effort—that I have completely expended myself and have left nothing on the course. The whole experience, from start to finish, awakens sleeping neurons in me like no other event. It makes me feel alive.

Lastly, a marathon is a great venue for meditation. The long run sweeps the cobwebs from my mind, and my focus becomes less obscured. I can clearly recall things from my past, good and bad, right and wrong. I may remember those people I should have helped and then make a mental note to do so the next time. In other words, a marathon allows me to get in touch with myself.

On the flip side, running can be noncerebral; that is, I do not have to focus on anything. All that is required is putting one foot in front of the other. It is automatic, pure muscle memory.

This is unlike our prehistoric ancestors who had to focus on running down an animal for food or to focus on running away from becoming food of a predator.

As an aside, an archeologist discovered the oldest known prehistoric human—a woman—in 1974. He found 40 percent of her skeleton at Hadar, a site of paleoanthropological excavations in the lower Awash River valley in the Afar region of Ethiopia. The archeologist named her "Lucy" after the Beatles' song, which was playing at the time of the discovery. Lucy lived 3.5 million years ago. Her catalogued name is "Afar location #288–1 (AL288–1)."

When archeologists find my bones in 3.5 million years, I wonder how they will catalogue me. Most likely, I will be unearthed in a Gulf Coast location. Remains of my running shoes will be on my bony feet. My favorite number is seven, so maybe an archeologist will discover me at location #7. Then, they will name and catalog me "Alabama Redneck Runner ALRR-GC7."

These were my wandering thoughts as I was trying to disavow that I had leukemia on a long, lonely car trip.

• • •

By the time I reached the city limits of Houston, it was early evening, although it had felt like evening the entire trip. Rain clouds had blocked all of the sun's light, making this trip that much more depressing.

I checked into the Houston Crowne Plaza Hotel, which the cancer center had recommended. The hotel was close to MD Anderson Cancer Center and provided free shuttle service. After checking in, I walked to Ruby Tuesday where I enjoyed a rib-eye steak dinner and a Beefeater gin martini, shaken with olives.

Back in my room after dinner, I called friends and family to let them know I had arrived and then went to bed. As I lay in bed, reality began to raise its ugly head. Denial had fueled this trip; now, I could not help but contemplate what tomorrow would convey.

I pushed myself to think positive thoughts. Like one of the doctors suggested, *Maybe I am just getting old.*

Similar to Dorothy on the yellow brick road, I was in search of my own Wizard, a Magician who would make all my wrongs right again. My final thought before falling asleep was, *I hope the MD Anderson Wizard has a solution that will get me back on the road to Boston.*

• • •

The next morning I boarded a shuttle bus at eight o'clock sharp. I was not the only one seeking an audience with the Wizard. The bus was laden with travelers on their way to the MD Anderson Cancer Center. I scrutinized the passengers as I worked my way down the aisle to a seat. I wondered, *Is there as much fear in my eyes as there is in theirs?*

On the bus, there were so many conversations going on at the same time. These conversations oh, so carefully avoided any topics of sickness. Just like me, these pursuers of the Wizard were attempting to take their minds off their fact-finding missions. We all had the big "C" and were in search of answers, of hope. Very few likely knew what was awaiting them, and some (like me) probably were hesitant to know. I just wanted the oncologist to tell me that I could run.

No one asked what the other one had, and no one volunteered that information. If I had not known better, I would have thought it was a tour bus to the Grand Canyon. An outside observer probably would not expect this to be a shuttle bus to a cancer center.

I reached an empty seat and quickly retired to my own special happy place. I tuned out my surroundings. I had plenty of time later to focus on leukemia and mortality. To do so then would have dislodged me from my carefully crafted denial.

I went to a place where I mentally felt comfortable. My thoughts were about simpler times, like when I grew up on a cattle ranch outside of a small Florida town named Bushnell. I attended South Sumter High School, and I was a member of the high school track team, although not because I was good at it. At school, for every sport we wanted to participate in, we had to sign up for a second one. (I mentioned that it was a small town; this was how the school ensured fully stocked sports teams.) I wanted to play baseball, so I ran track as well. Not being good at track, I would later replace it with basketball.

One of my regrets is having lost contact with so many high school friends. Unfortunately, our lives pass so quickly that it is sometimes years—decades even—before we appreciate how important those relationships are.

• • •

"Sir, sir, we are at MD Anderson."

I was so absorbed in my daydream that I was unaware that we had arrived. I looked around. Everyone had exited the bus. I thanked the driver and tipped him before stepping off.

I hesitantly entered what seemed like the dungeon of doom; the doors to the MD Anderson Cancer Center seemed like the gates of hell. People talk about their lives flashing before their eyes just before dying, but mine did so as I stepped inside the cancer center. Exposed like a gaping wound were memories of every disparaging comment I had made and of all the people I had wronged. I was amazed at how many of those instances I recalled at a moment's notice. This must have been God's way of reminding me that I needed lots of remodeling. I would have no shortage of topics to talk about to the priest during my next confession. It occurred to me that I should not procrastinate that meeting.

I believe that God will forgive us our sins if we repent, but I am not sure if the people we have hurt will forgive us. The Bible teaches us that forgiveness is a Christian act, but even then, people are reluctant to do so. Therefore, I would simply have to rely on God's forgiveness and let the chips fall where they may with those I have wronged.

• • •

After getting my bearings and taking a few shaky breaths, I entered one of the many elevators and pressed the button for the eighth floor. Reaching my destination, I emerged and walked to the registration desk, where a friendly smile greeted me. A voice behind the smile said, "Good morning. How may I help you?"

"Hi, I'm Phillip Fields. I have an appointment with Dr. Keating."

"Please sign the registration book."

As I did so, the woman behind the smile handed me a stack of papers. "This is a packet of information for you to read and sign. Return them to my desk when you have finished. You may have a seat in the lounge, and someone will come to get you shortly."

The waiting room would become a familiar place during the next three days. Not having brought a friend or a good book, I had plenty of free time to indulge in reminiscence. Although I now had a packet of papers to look over and sign. There were various forms with an ID number printed at the top of each page. They were obviously ready for me. My ID number was 737908. I speculated, *Am I the 737,908ᵗʰ patient they have seen with leukemia?*

The first two forms were "Privacy Practices" and "Information Disclosure." The third form was a bit more disconcerting: "Consent to Diagnosis and Treatment." I was prepared for a diagnosis, but not for treatment. I deliberated over that statement. *Surely, things are not so bad that the oncologist is going to admit me and begin treatment during this trip. I need time to prepare, not only mentally but also physically. I have a cat named Speedi back home that needs my care. Then there is work. Who is going to give my lectures?*

I hesitated, my pen hovering above the paper, but after a moment, I signed that form, too.

The last form was "Permission to Collect and Store Tissue Samples." As I signed that form, I chuckled to myself, thinking, *If they want my body organs, they will have to get in line. I am already a body donor at the medical school where I teach human anatomy and embryology.*

Having completed that task, I considered the fact that I was now a statistic. I had lost my former identity and had become Patient #737908.

I had no sooner returned the forms to the receptionist and sat back down when I heard, "Phillip Fields?"

"Yes."

"Please follow me."

That simple exchange of words became familiar over the next three days.

A young girl in a pink smock, a volunteer, led me to an office to discuss my health insurance. A woman behind a desk greeted me with a friendly smile before we got down to the business of confirming my health coverage. After a brief period of silence, while she entered my information into her computer, she looked up at me. "Your insurance will cover everything except the $400 copay for clinical tests. You can pay with cash, or by check or credit card."

My eyebrows furrowed in confusion as I said, "I checked with Blue Cross Blue Shield before this trip and was told that all expenses would be paid. Would you mind calling them to clarify this?"

She kindly made the call.

Later, while begrudgingly writing a check for $400, I thought about all those patients I had seen earlier that morning. *Many probably do not have medical insurance as good as I have through my university.* Over the years, I have learned that I do not have to look far to find someone whose situation is worse than my own.

As soon as I returned to the waiting room, the receptionist again called me to her desk. She handed me another mountain of forms to fill out. At the top of each page was typed my new identity, #737908. These forms contained blanks for personal information, prior surgeries, and medical issues about my parents and me. One question really caught my attention: Do you have a living will? Not only did I not have a living will, I did not have any type of will. I indicated so on the form, making a mental note to myself, *Under the circumstances, I should work on having a will prepared when I get back home.* (If you do not have a living will, I recommend that you read the book, *It's OK to Die*, by Monica Williams-Murphy M.D. and Kristian Murphy. This incredible book discusses the need for a living will and things to consider when creating one.)

There is nothing like a health crisis to remind me to take care of important issues. After all, this is one of the top leukemia centers in the country. I was not there for a common cold.

Now, I felt even more anxious and alone. I closed my eyes and reminisced about better times, when leukemia did not encumber my running, like after graduating from high school in 1965. That was when I began running four to five miles a day. I soon learned that this activity afforded me a certain level of peace. It quickly became therapeutic—a place I could withdraw to in order to relieve stress. I had not yet developed a passion for running marathons. Soon, that would change.

CHAPTER 4
First Marathon

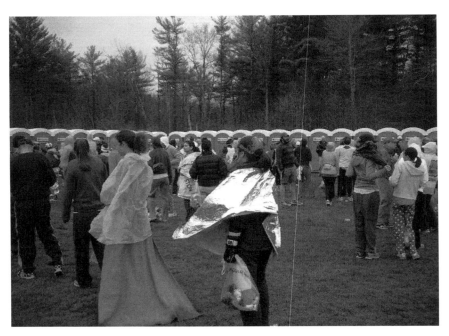

Lines at the Port-o-Lets (Boston Marathon 2004)

"Etiquette is the fine tuning of education."
Nadine Daher[6]

Several years after moving to Mobile, Alabama, I read about the Pleasure Island Marathon in Gulf Shores. I had never run a marathon, but I was immediately intrigued; 26.2 miles sounded like a good challenge. When I signed up for this marathon, I went through a spectrum of sensations: excitement, anxiety, and then fear. I felt similar emotions on my first day of junior varsity football practice (**Chapter Related Memory: The Football Helmet**. The story is at the end of the chapter).

My knowledge of a marathon consisted of the mileage, and that was it. I had no idea how to train for or run one. Of course, that did not matter since there was not much time for training; the race was less than a month away. I reasoned, *The distance is less than six times my daily run. I will just run slower than normal in order to complete the race.* At the time, my strategy seemed foolproof. Needless to say, my strategy was foolish. I look back now and think, *You idiot!*

Because it was my first road race and I did not know what to expect, I arrived early. I saw several long lines of runners. I approached a runner and asked, "What is this line for?"

He responded, "The bathroom."

Needing to go, I got behind him.

"So, what is the building at the front of the line?" I asked, making some chitchat.

The runner looked at me as if I were some sort of space alien from another planet. He replied with a scoff, "It's a port-o-let."

I could tell from the tone in his voice that he would like to have added, "Dummy."

I looked at the little blue building with curiosity. After the fifth grade, I began spending my summers working in watermelon, cucumber, tomato, or bell pepper fields. Then later, I worked in orange groves, herded cattle, and had various part-time construction jobs. There was always a bathroom to use, or a tree or building to go behind. There was never a port-o-let.

It seems incredulous, even improbable, that at thirty-seven years old this was my first one. I have since entered close to a thousand port-o-lets. My first marathon would be full of many new experiences.

After relieving myself of excess fluid, I looked around inside the port-o-let and thought, *That is strange. The low sink on the left side has no water hookup. So, how am I supposed to wash my hands?* I exited without doing so.

After my introduction to the port-o-let, I worked my way to the packet pickup. I retrieved my racing bib and watched how others pinned theirs to their running shorts or shirt. I had a heck of a time getting that bib pinned on straight and to the center of my shirt. I reasoned that if I pinned the bid on straight, the other runners would not view me as a novice. Before too long, I would learn that that particular detail did not matter.

With the bib perfectly pinned to my shirt, my next stop was the front of the starting line. Wow, did I ever feel out of place! Runners were wearing color-coordinated outfits with brightly colored running shoes fresh out of the box. My shorts and shirt were mismatched, and my shoes were old and dirty. It was as though I had shown up to a dance in slacks and a sport shirt, only to realize upon entering that the event was a formal ball.

Runners at the starting line were talking as if they knew what they were doing. There was a strange conversation about things called "mile splits" and "negative splits." Some runners were talking about how fast they planned to go through the first half of the marathon. I heard others predicting their marathon finishing time based on a previously run 10K race. Somehow, these runners, who seemed almost like professionals to my novice ears, knew how that information would predict their finishing time for this marathon.

I overheard a couple of runners talking about how fast they had run their last marathon. They boasted that their finishing time had qualified them for something called the Boston Marathon. At the time, I had no idea what any of that meant. They may as well have been speaking Greek.

When the race official announced that there was one minute to the start of the race, runners around me began pressing buttons on their strange-looking watches. I looked at my own wrist; I had a Timex that gave only the time. Of course, that did not matter. I had not calculated what pace would give me a particular finishing time. Heck, I did not even have a finishing time in mind. I was simply testing the water.

As I stood at the starting line and listened for the pistol shot that would announce the beginning of the race, I felt like I might throw up. It was as if 10,000 Monarch butterflies took flight at one time inside my stomach. I contemplated leaving. Before I could decide, the gun went off: I was committed.

When the marathon started, I just stood there frozen in place. Runners were blowing past me as if this was a 100-yard dash. They were elbowing and cursing me as they went by: "Either run or get out of the race." Then another said, "If you aren't a good runner, line up at the back."

Thus, I learned my first lesson: It is not proper etiquette to line up at the front of the race if you are not one of the fast runners. I made a mental note to start keeping such revelations in a journal.

Eventually, all of those color-coordinated, fancy-watch-wearing runners brushed past me, and I was among runners who looked more like me. I was now in my comfort zone. My plan was to run slower than my daily running pace of seven minutes. I reached mile 2 in sixteen minutes, which was a comfortable eight-minute pace. That is also when I began to panic; I had not brought anything to drink.

Shortly after that fright, I saw a table beside the road where volunteers were handing out Styrofoam cups filled with water. (Today's health-conscious racing community only uses paper cups.)

I added another entry to my mental journal: It is not proper etiquette to pause in the middle of a water stop to drink. Again, runners were crashing into me, cursing me. "Hey, watch what you're doing!"

"Get out of the middle of the road to drink!"

Race brochures have stopped referring to these as "water stops" and now call them "aid stations." I guess they are trying to get rid of the subtle message in the word "stop". (This obviously has not worked. After years of running marathons, I still see runners stopping in the middle of aid stations to drink.)

Feeling good at mile 10, my confidence grew. I thought, *This is going to be a lot easier than I anticipated.* That is when the silence became evident. At the beginning of the race, everyone was talking and laughing. Now, the only sounds were those of feet hitting the pavement and the heavy, measured breathing of the runners.

Still feeling good at mile 12, I decided to increase my pace. I ran miles 13 and 14 in fifteen minutes, a seven-and-a-half-minute pace. I began passing many runners and I recalled reading about age group awards. I imagined myself getting one in my first marathon. No, my first race, period. My thoughts began to wander. I saw myself crossing the finish line and later, the race director calling me up on stage to receive my award. In my mind, I sheepishly grinned and waved to the clapping racers below. Maybe those front-of-the-pack runners would remember me and be impressed.

My adrenaline was flowing, and I wondered what the trophy would look like. So intoxicating was the mental image of receiving a trophy that I began to calculate, thinking to myself, *If I increase my pace another thirty seconds per mile, how much will I improve my finish time?*

I ran miles 15 and 16 in fourteen minutes, which was a seven-minute pace. I can assure you that the amount of pain suffered by that blunder was increased exponentially more than my preconceived improvement in my finish time.

I ran mile 17 in nine minutes and mile 18 in eleven minutes. I did not even realize my pace was slowing, although it did seem like the mile markers were getting further apart.

By mile 19, my brain was in oxygen debt. It was impossible to calculate my pace any longer using mile markers and a watch that only gave the time of day. I made another mental note or, really, a promise to myself that, if I did this again, I would get a watch with more buttons on it.

By mile 20, I was done. It hurt to walk, much less run. I never realized so many body parts could hurt at the same time. My thighs, calves, feet, neck, abdominal muscles, and shoulders ached. I could feel blisters on my feet and chaffing in areas that I never realized rubbed together. Even the tips of my big toes were throbbing, although at the time I was not sure why.

I had never before felt such physical stress and thought, *Maybe I am dying and should stop.*

I approached a volunteer who was handing out water and asked, "Can I get a ride to the finish line?"

"Sure," he said. "Right after the last runner passes and we pack things up. There is an army cot under that tree that you can lie on while you're waiting."

I am not sure how long I napped. On wakening and seeing runners still going by the water stop, six miles no longer seemed that far. I got up and made my way back to the road. I started with a slight jog, and soon, I was running again. I finished in four hours and thirty-five minutes (4:35). I was happy not being last; heck, I was happy to be at the finish line (even though I did not win an age group award).

I am glad I got up and finished the marathon. Otherwise, it would likely have been my last attempt to run one. Had I quit, I would not have experienced the exhilaration of having run farther than ever before. In fact, 26.2 miles was five times farther than my longest run, even if I did briefly stop to take a nap. Had I not gotten off that cot and finished that marathon, today I would be looking back and asking myself, *What would be different if I had failed to finish that marathon?* Keep this in mind as you read where I go from that moment at the Pleasure Island Marathon. I know that I have thought about this.

While limping to my car, I felt good about my accomplishment. In that moment, I was experiencing my first true runner's high. My euphoria quickly disappeared, and in its place, a runners low appeared as I threw up what little fluid remained in my stomach. This resulted in my last mental note of the day: *It is better to park close to the finish line. Hobbling this far back to the car is not fun.*

While driving home, I pulled off the road several times because of cramps in my calves and feet. During one of those stops, I promised myself that I would never run another marathon. I forgot about the promise five days later when I was again able to walk down the stairs normally rather than going down backwards. I began looking for another marathon to run. I felt confident that things would be different for the next marathon. That first marathon taught me a lot about running marathons, things I would use for years to come.

When I told friends, "I am going to run another marathon," they asked, "Why would you want to punish yourself like that again?"

The only answer I could summon was, "To improve my time." Nevertheless, the reason was more than that. Pushing myself through the pain was invigorating. I cannot accurately describe the experience except to say that I felt alive. Besides, I have always enjoyed a good challenge, and my first marathon had thrown down a gauntlet that I could not just let lie there.

It was sort of like the game my brother Michael and I played as kids. On our cattle ranch, the bull pasture had an electric fence around the inside of the barbed wire fence. This prevented the bull from getting among the cows when we did not want him to.

Whenever a friend visited, we went into the pasture and lined up in front of the electric fence. On the count of three, we all grabbed the fence with both hands. The idea was to see who could hang on the longest. I never won, but I kept competing, determinedly grabbing that electric fence and envisioning myself as the last man standing. We must have looked rather silly to the bull.

Chapter Related Memory: The Football Helmet

*Excitement, anxiety, and then fear. I felt similar emo-
tions on my first day of junior varsity football practice.*

I was thirteen years old and in the ninth grade. When I entered the gymnasium, the other junior varsity football players were dressed and heading out to the football field. The football gear was in various piles in the middle of the gym floor. There was a pile with helmets, a pile with shirts, and a pile with pants. Several other piles had various types of padding. We were required to purchase our own shoes. I had not done so yet and showed up in tennis shoes, black and white high tops—Keds I believe. Coach Grinstaff was on his way out the door and yelled back at me to dress quickly and get outside. I was in a state of frozen animation while staring at those piles of strange objects. I had no idea where to start and considered my options. I could stay or leave.

The varsity players were beginning to dress for their prac-
tice. Jackie Huggins (a friend), said, "What are you doing, Fields? You better get dressed like the coach said."

"I have no idea how to put this stuff on." I responded.

A good friend and sympathetic to my plight, Jackie showed me how the equipment was properly worn. Just as I was strapping on the last of the pads, the coach returned to see what was tak-
ing me so long. Everyone in the gym heard his booming voice: "Fields! Get out to the field immediately, or you will be running laps until the cows come home." Living on a cattle ranch, his comment had meaning. The coach then glared at me. "What in the hell are you doing? Get that equipment on correctly and get outside."

Jackie had helped me strap the shoulder pads around my waist and the hip pads around my shoulders. The gear did not look or feel right, but I was clueless. The varsity players enjoyed a good laugh at my expense.

After practice, the coach introduced me to my first serious running, although I arrived home before the cows came up to the barn for feeding.

That was also my last day of junior varsity football. Mom was the county nurse and came to the second day of practice to perform player physicals. Seeing me among the players, she would not sign my release form so I could play. Mom was very protective. My reaction to this was indifference—the football helmet did not fit me anyway.

CHAPTER 5

First Love

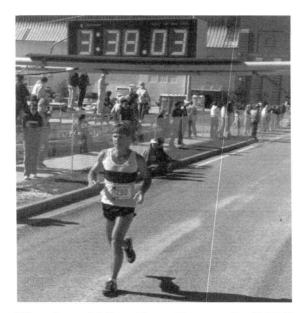

Blue Angel Marathon, Pensacola (1986)

A first love is something that lasts forever in your heart.
It's something that marks you.

Elodie Yung[7]

My first marathon, the Pleasure Island Marathon (1984), was the genesis of a love affair, the birth of my passion. That marathon opened a door to an unknown area of my inner self, a place I can only experience when I push beyond my pain threshold. Little did I know, as I sat in the waiting room at MD Anderson Cancer Center (January 2008), attempting to run a marathon with leukemia would totally redefine my pain threshold.

My name cut through the air, disrupting my recollection.

"Phillip Fields?"

"Yes."

"Please follow me."

I followed the girl in the pink smock to an examining room. After a short wait, an official-looking entourage of white-coated doctors entered. The group included one of the top blood oncologists in the country, Dr. Michael Keating. They affectionately refer to these doctors as a HemOnc—one who specializes in hematology and oncology. Very quickly, I could tell that one of his skills was in his bedside manner. His demeanor immediately put me at ease, a great feat considering my state of mind.

He was a stately looking man with a full white beard. He reminded me of Gandalf the Grey in *The Lord of the Rings*. All that was missing was a magical staff. Fittingly, magic was what I sought—a supernatural solution for my ailment, a remedy that would get me back on the road to Boston.

"Hi, I'm Dr. Keating. These are my associates."

"Hi, I'm Dr. Fields. I am here because whatever I have is interfering with my passion, running marathons. I was training for my third Boston marathon when my running took an unexpected turn for the worse."

I wondered if I had been too abrupt. Regardless, I wanted him to know that running was extremely important to me, as if that was going to make a difference.

It did not seem to faze him, though. "So you have qualified for Boston? You must be a good runner!"

I shook my head. "Not really. I am just average for those at Boston, but I still love running them. I need your help so that I can get back to my training and back to Boston." I needed him to understand the importance of my words, but I could hear the pleading in my voice. I felt embarrassed.

In a soft, calming voice he responded, "We have looked over the clinical records you sent us, and you definitely have leukemia." He then described the routine for the next three days. "We will be evaluating numerous lymphocyte cell markers in order to determine the type of leukemia you have and how aggressive it is."

Many of the cell markers were the same as those evaluated in Mobile; some were different. MD Anderson would conduct most of the tests, although an analytical lab in California would assay one key cell marker. Coincidentally, that marker was the same one the pathologist in Mobile had failed to obtain.

Dr. Keating wished me good luck and exited as quickly as he had appeared. I would not see him again until the third day.

Back in the waiting room, I sat and wondered, *What did Dr. Keating mean by "good luck"? Did he mean "good luck" with ever running the Boston Marathon again? Or, was he wishing me "good luck" because of my leukemia? Was it a foreboding "good luck," as in wishing me well because I am going to need it? Where had he placed the emphasis?*

Before I had time to get comfortable, a voice interrupted my thoughts.

"Phillip Fields?"

"Yes."

"Please follow me."

The volunteer in the pink smock escorted me to an examination room. A nurse entered, and like everyone else I had met so far, she was smiling as she asked, "How are you today?"

I made a weak attempt at comic relief, "I am like the groundskeeper at the cemetery: 'Another day above ground.'"

I am not sure why I said that. Maybe I hoped that by making fun of the situation, the eventual diagnosis would not be so bad. Alternatively, maybe I was attempting to prove I was strong and not afraid.

My humor did not make an impression on the nurse or alleviate my fears.

"Please stand on the scale so I can get your weight," the nurse said. As I did so, I again attempted to be funny, "One at a time please," as if the scales were talking.

Without so much as a chuckle, she called out the numbers as she wrote in her chart. "Your weight is 175 pounds."

While I stood on the scale, she extended the bar and brought it down on top of my head. "Your height is five feet, eight inches."

I looked at the nurse in confusion. "Wait, that can't be right. I have always been five feet, ten inches. That is what my high school basketball coach listed as my height."

She remeasured. "No, you are five feet, eight inches."

Before I had time to give this new revelation much thought, I was ushered to a chair. There, the nurse placed a thermometer in my mouth and wrapped a blood pressure cuff around my arm. She started to make small talk, "So, I hear you run marathons. How many have you run?"

I hate when people do that—stick an instrument in my mouth and then ask me a question. For example, the dentist sticks a mirror, a suction tube, and a scraper in my mouth and then begins asking about my family or school.

The nurse again called out the numbers. "Your temperature is 97.8—normal. Your blood pressure is 116/70, and your pulse rate is 75."

I briefly mulled over that last number: *My pulse rate is a bit high; it is normally around 55–60. It could be elevated due to my knowledge about what is getting ready to happen.*

The next routine had become all too familiar during the past three months. As expected, the nurse began methodically laying out serum vials. I could feel my heart rate increase even more. (By the way, I hate needles, and I always have.)

She tied a rubber strap around my biceps, pinching my skin in the process. Next, she rubbed the front of my elbow joint with alcohol and inserted a needle into one of my veins. I have learned that this final procedure is less painful if the nurse inserts the needle after the alcohol has dried. She did not do so.

The lab would use my blood to determine blood counts and to evaluate the function of my thyroid gland, liver, and kidneys. After she filled the last vial, the volunteer in the pink smock escorted me back to the waiting room.

Although everyone I had encountered so far at MD Anderson had been friendly, it was a terribly depressing place. Considering all the horror stories I had heard growing up, this was not a place people visited and left.

Having failed to bring a friend or a good book, remembrances were my only defense against thinking about where I was or why I was here.

• • •

I certainly remember everything about my first marathon. I liken that event to my first love. You see, I remember every detail about her, as well.

Barbara Jean Milton was her full name, and her beauty was breathtaking. The first time I met her was at my junior college graduation (1967). I had no idea she existed, but she apparently knew who I was. She walked up with a smile and handed me a bag of chocolate chip cookies that she had baked herself.

"Congratulations on your graduation," she said smoothly, her smile never faltering.

Like a dummy, I just stood there looking at that bag of cookies. Not knowing what to say, I eventually thanked her and walked off to visit with friends. Back then, I was as clueless about women as I was about my first marathon. (Of course, I still am.)

Driving home after the graduation ceremony, I could not stop thinking about the girl with the cookies. If there is such a thing as love at first sight, I had just experienced it.

I finally asked my mother, "Who was the girl that gave me the cookies?"

Mom was the county health nurse and knew everyone. True to form, she provided not only her name (Barbara "Babs" Jean Milton) but also details about Babs and her family. This conversation was a bit unusual, Mom had nothing negative to say about Babs.

• • •

There were times when having a county health nurse for a mother was detrimental to the romantic lives of my brother Michael and me. Mom was protective and possessive of her sons. She would come up with the most horrific stories to discourage us in our pursuits, which quickly killed our interest in a specific girl.

When Michael was sixteen, he went on a date with a girl that Mom did not approve of. She would not tell Michael directly that she disapproved of the girl. Instead, she came home from work on Monday with a quart jar full of roundworm, Ascaris lumbricoides. These are one of the vilest looking parasitic worms.

Mom showed the jar to Michael, saying, "These were passed from the girl you went out with Saturday." Having grown up with Mom's vivid descriptions of medical events, we were well aware what "passed from" meant. Mom later confessed that the worms were not from Michael's date, but Michael could not bring himself to ask the girl out again.

• • •

Mom apparently tired of my questions about Babs and encouraged me to call her. I remember how strange that seemed to me and I thought, *How unusual. Mom actually approves of Babs enough to encourage me to ask her out. What, no jar of worms, no story of a puss-oozing sore or a history of head lice?* Then I wondered if mom was using some form of reverse psychology on me, to confuse me by appearing to like Babs, hoping I would not call her.

I eventually worked up enough courage to make the phone call. There has been no other time that I have been that nervous calling a girl on the phone. I had already surmised there was something extraordinarily special about Babs; I did not want to squander my opportunity.

This happened over forty years ago, so I can recall only a few details about that phone conversation. I have never been good at small talk, so I am sure that I sounded like an idiot.

I learned that she was only a junior at Wildwood High School and that she was Baptist.

There was an awkward period of silence after this last revelation. I could not think of anything to say as I mulled this disclosure over in my mind. I thought, *Mom has to know this. We are Catholic, yet she still encouraged this encounter. Surely, her parents are not going to allow me to date their daughter. What if they do and I find that I am really in love with her? Religion will doom our relationship before it begins.*

"Are you still there?" Babs asked.

I responded, "Yes. How do you know me, and why were you at my graduation?"

"I read about your accomplishments in 4-H livestock judging, and I saw you at the county fair."

I realized that she was talking about events that had happened more than three to four years ago. I tried to remember if I had seen her at any 4-H event, but I could not remember.

She continued, "My mother drove me to the graduation ceremony so that I could meet you."

I then remembered how I seemingly had rejected her that evening and thought, *It is amazing she is talking to me. She must really like me.* I could feel my heart beating. Falling in love is an incredible yet indescribable feeling. Once you feel it, you never mistake it as merely a passing interest in someone.

This was back when there were party lines if you had a phone. I could hear someone picking up and putting down the receiver as Babs and I were talking. Mom came into the kitchen a moment later. "Okay, that's enough. It's time to tell her good-bye," Mom said.

I told Babs I had to get off the phone, said goodbye, and hung up. Then it hit me, *You idiot! You did not ask her for a date!* I immediately tried to call her back, but the phone line was in use. I eventually reached her, and we began what turned into a beautiful relationship, one that blossomed because of a small bag of chocolate chip cookies.

We dated for a little over two years while I attended the University of Florida. We began discussing marriage and when would be the best time to do so. I was graduating from The University of Florida and was going to Texas A&M University for graduate school. Babs was graduating from high school and wanted to go to college. We agreed that it was best to wait to get married until she finished college. That seemed like a lifetime to wait.

Neither of us brought up the subject of religion. I guess we were both afraid to do so. I was more than happy to put off that discussion.

Just before leaving for Texas A&M University, I learned that she was seeing someone else. When I confronted her, she calmly told me that she did not want to see me anymore. My dream of spending a lifetime with someone I loved simply evaporated. I have often wondered, *Was the religion issue too much for her to cope with? Did I make a mistake by not talking about that issue early in our relationship?* These questions haunted me for years.

I had never lost anyone I loved, and I had no idea that something could hurt so much. Because of the pain from losing Babs, I promised myself that I would never allow myself to fall in love again. Yet years later, beautiful memories of the time that I had spent with Babs replaced the hurt. I did love again, just as I ran a marathon again.

I have heard people talk about two things they never forget: For some it is their first love, and for others it is their first marathon. Having experienced and done poorly at both, I agree with them.

My first love, like my first marathon, was not a total failure, and I was confident that I had learned ways to improve myself because of both of them. I concluded that the next time I would do better to ensure an improved outcome. Yet, would I?

CHAPTER 6

Worst Decision

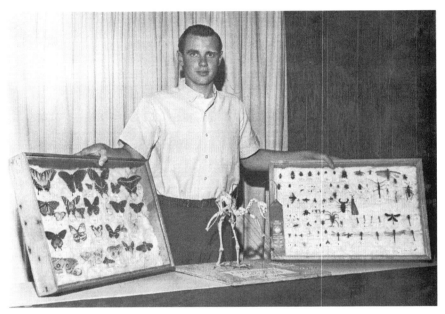

4-H Entomology Collection and Chicken Skeleton (1963)

Love never dies,
as long as there is someone who remembers.
Leo Buscaglia[8]

For nearly forty years, I had managed to block memories of Babs. Now, as I sat in the waiting room at MD Anderson Cancer Center in January 2008, these memories were resurfacing from all directions, like ghosts in a haunted house in New Orleans. I am sure it had something to do with the environment, this "dungeon of death," as I called it.

The next memory was the worst of them all: the reason I had pushed away all memories of the woman with whom I had hoped to spend my life. It was a moment in time that I would love to have the chance to go back to and do differently.

It was October 1970, and I was in my second year of graduate school at Texas A&M University. My birthday is October 17, and I received a large package in the mail from Babs' mother. Seeing the return address reopened a wound that had just begun to heal. It was a birthday cake with a card wishing me well. I was stunned and stared at the cake and card in disbelief. I asked myself, *Why did she send me a cake? I did not think she particularly cared for me since I was Catholic.*

My brother and I ate the cake anyway.

Three days after the cake arrived, I got a phone call from Babs. I was stupefied, so much so that I was unable to make an intelligent decision in the minutes that followed.

She told me about her college and that she had decided to become a dental hygienist. She talked about the newest style in girls' clothing—miniskirts—and said she was sure I would love seeing her in one. Then, like lightning out of nowhere in a cloudless sky, she asked if we could get back together. I was confused. This was unexpected, painful, and wonderful at the same time. Yet, the pain from losing her the first time still felt fresh in my memory. This prevented me from screaming, *Yes, yes, God yes.* Instead, I heard myself saying, "I'm sorry, but too much water has passed under that bridge, and I am not sure I still love you."

After my stupid, idiotic comment, there was nothing left to say other than goodbye. As I hung the phone up, tears filled my eyes. I hoped she would call back; I was too proud or stupid to do so myself. She did not, and I never saw her again. (I recently learned that she passed away in 2011 after a two-year battle with cancer. I will never have an opportunity to tell her that I never stopped loving her.)

• • •

Thankfully, the sound of my name pulled me out of that painful memory.

"Phillip Fields?"

"Yes."

"Please follow me."

The volunteer led me back to the nursing station that I had just left. The nurse had forgotten to collect a urine sample. A simple mistake, yet I felt as uneasy as I had when Dr. Butler was collecting that bone marrow sample. An "Oops" is not what I want to hear when it involves my health, even if it only involves peeing in a cup.

I was only half a day into my visit at the cancer center, and I felt numb, or maybe mindless, like one of the "walkers" in *The Walking Dead*. Of course, they are in a never-ending search for humans to feed on; I was in search of answers. So far, I had only written a check for $400, filled out countless forms, met the oncologist, had vital measurements taken, had blood drawn, and lastly, provided a urine sample.

Now, I was in search of food. Apparently, I was not the only one in search of a meal. A spider crawled across the wall in the waiting room. This was not one of those tiny jumping spiders either; it was huge. If I were into interpreting signs, I probably would have made something sinister out of that occurrence. I chose not to indulge in the paranormal. Instead, it was just a strange sight to see in a hospital (**Chapter Related Memory: Pet Spider**. The story is at the end of the chapter).

After lunch, I returned to an almost vacant waiting room and thought, *Maybe they do all of the testing in the mornings and let people go home in the afternoon. I hope I am through for the day.*

• • •

"Phillip Fields?"

"Yes."

This was a new face. As ready as I was for this exhausting first day to end, I asked myself, almost annoyed, *What does she want?* I immediately assumed a defensive posture, the sort of pose I strike when a salesperson approaches me.

She introduced herself and said, "I'm in charge of housing arrangements for patients seeking treatment at MD Anderson." She handed me a brochure and continued, "This will describe the various types of patient housing that are available."

I did not say anything. This was the first time that someone said "treatment" on this trip. Moreover, I was hearing it from a person in charge of housing, not a doctor. I was even more anxious and more than slightly annoyed at the timing of this encounter. I wanted to say, *Shouldn't this discussion occur at the end of the three days, not on the first day of my visit?* For once, though, I kept my mouth shut.

She described the housing for patients receiving chemotherapy, "We have apartments for those who require only a few months of treatment. There is also housing for those requiring a stay of six months or longer. The rooms came equipped with a kitchen and a room for guests or family members."

Six months or longer? I thought without speaking. She must have seen the shocked expression on my face, because she back-pedaled, "Of course, your treatment might not take six months." It was too late. Her comment had already set off a chain reaction in my nerve synapses. My central nervous system was releasing neu-rotransmitters as my brain attempted to translate her comments.

She continued with more mind-numbing information; I tuned her out. I did not "go" anywhere in particular or have rec-ollections about Babs, bugs, or bathrooms. I simply stopped lis-tening. Her speech had become nothing more than white noise.

An unmistakable silence broke my concentration on a pot-ted plant. The woman had finished talking. She gave me her card, said to contact her if I had any questions, and walked away.

"Questions!" I scoffed, not realizing that I had said it aloud.

She turned around, "Yes?"

"Nothing, I was just thinking out loud."

I wanted to scream. As the only one left in the waiting room, I thought about actually doing so. I refrained since I did not want them to transfer me from the cancer ward to the psych ward. Instead, I again stared at that potted plant and contemplated what just happened: *A woman drops in out of nowhere, briefly describes housing for patients requiring treatment, and abruptly leaves. This seems so premature. There are no results yet. They have not determined how serious my leukemia is, and there has been no discussion with the oncologist about treatment.*

"Phillip Fields?"

It was the volunteer in the pink smock again.

"You are through for the day. They want you back at 9:00 tomorrow morning."

I practically sprinted from the building. Once outside, Houston's traffic exhaust replaced the noxious smell of the cancer center. The smog smelled wonderful.

On the shuttle bus back to the hotel, I was the lone passenger. I stared blankly out the window as we drove through the MD Anderson Medical Complex, which seemed endless. There was a building for every major health issue: lung, heart, brain, cancer, and kidney. As I just learned, there was even housing for patients and their families during treatment. This was a city within the city of Houston.

I arrived back at the hotel by early afternoon, and since it was too early for dinner, I decided to nap. I lay on my back and watched the ceiling fan. Like those fan blades, there was too much swirling around in my brain to nap. My first day at MD Anderson had been nothing more than filling out papers, giving blood, and drowning in a tangle of memories—some good and some sad. However, the day's events had accomplished one thing: They had systematically dislodged me from my comfort zone, my repudiation of having leukemia. The final shove was that housing representative. Thanks to her I wondered, *When will treatment begin? Can I receive chemotherapy at The Mitchell Cancer Institute in Mobile? If I have to come to Houston, the housing at MD Anderson does not allow pets. What will I do with my cat, Speedi? How is this going to affect my job?*

I enjoy having structure in my life, and all of the organization that I had nurtured over the years was rapidly turning into a shambles. My secure world was slowly disintegrating before my eyes. In its place, a new one was evolving.

Chapter Related Memory: Pet Spider

A spider just crawled across the wall in the waiting room.

As a ten-year-old sixth-grader, I was an amateur entomologist. This was one of my 4-H projects. I spent hours in the yard and pasture catching bugs and euthanizing them in a chloroform jar. I mounted them in large wooden boxes with a glass lid and a cotton-covered floor. I organized the bugs according to their scientific name and order. There were beetles (order Coleoptera), scorpions (order Scorpiones), spiders (order Araneae), and moths and butterflies (order Lepidoptera), just to name a few of them.

I probably looked ridiculous to our bull as I was running across the pasture and swatting at unseen objects with a butterfly net, not to mention what the neighbors must have thought.

Growing up on a cattle ranch in Central Florida, there was no shortage of Araneae (spiders). One weekend I caught a large black widow spider. She had that unmistakable red hourglass pattern on her jet-black undercarriage. I considered her quite a beauty. I placed her and her egg pod inside a glass display case. My brother used this case to show his honeybees at the 4-H county fair.

That Monday, I proudly took the spider to school for show-and-tell. I was excited as I exited the car at school with my pet. I thought, *This is going to be the best show-and-tell ever. It is going to be neat watching the egg pod hatch.*

Immediately after I entered the classroom, the teacher exited the classroom. The principal called Mom and asked her to come retrieve my pet and me. The principal gave me a note to give Mom. It said something about my being a disturbed child and needing psychological counseling. After years of these sorts of occurrences, Mom knew better. I got the day off from school, and Mom assured the principal the spider would not return.

So, what happened to my spider? Well, the display case had small slits in the top for air. The slits were too small for the adult spider to exit, but not for the babies. An egg pod can hatch as many as 200 offspring. I came home from school to find baby black widow spiders crawling all over the display case, my desk, and my bedroom wall. I got out a can of Raid, but I spared the spiders that were still in the case. I took them to a woodpile behind the barn and released them into the wild.

I guess it was a good thing they did not allow me to keep the spider at school. Had those baby spiders found their way out of the display case inside the classroom, the school might not have let me return.

CHAPTER 7
Brothers

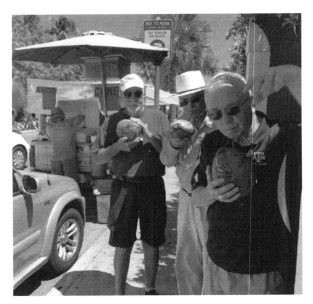

Left to Right: Tim, Michael, and Russell (Key West 2015)

I sought my soul, but my soul I could not see.
I sought my God, but my God eluded me.
I sought my brother and I found all three.

William Blake[9]

Unable to sleep after my first day at MD Anderson, I closed my eyes and thought back to my childhood and my big brother. I am four years younger than Michael is, and it seems like I have spent my entire life attempting to walk in his footprints. Some kids end up with psychological problems because their parents expect them to live up to standards of an older sibling. They present the younger child with a yardstick that they are unable to equal. For me, this was not an issue. I chose to emulate my big brother.

For example, in high school, Michael joined the 4-H club, so I did too. Michael was elected to a state office in the 4-H club (Parliamentarian), and I was later elected State Reporter. One of Michael's 4-H projects was raising bees; one of mine was collecting bugs (similar projects, but my bugs were dead and did not sting me).

In high school, Michael joined the Key Club, and the members elected him District Lieutenant Governor. When I was old enough, I joined the Key Club, and the members elected me District Lieutenant Governor. His tenure was extremely productive; mine was mediocre.

After graduating from high school (1965) and then junior college (1967), I joined my brother at the University of Florida. We roomed together while Michael worked on his master's degree. In 1969, he went to Texas A&M University for his PhD in reproductive physiology. I also ended up at Texas A&M University after graduating from the University of Florida (1969). We were again roommates as I worked on a master's degree in meat science. Michael completed his PhD and began working at The University of Florida in the Animal Science Department. Years later (1976), I graduated with a PhD in biochemistry from Texas A&M University and trailed after him to the University of Florida to get a postdoctorate degree at the College of Medicine. We again lived together. Our classic brotherly relationship never lost its appeal. We both loved every moment.

In 1980, I accepted a faculty position at the University of South Alabama, College of Medicine in Mobile, Alabama. I teach human anatomy and human embryology to medical students and conduct research in reproductive biology.

I was not through tagging along after Michael. We had taken different paths, yet we both ended up working on the biochemistry and physiology of the same hormone, called "relaxin." Thus, it was only natural that we would collaborate on research projects. Brothers, through and through. (As a side note, "relaxin" is no typo. Although Michael and I have done a lot of relaxing during our scientific careers, this hormone is relaxin, with no "g." The discoverer of the hormone so named it because it causes a dilation of the cervix and a relaxation of the pelvic ligaments during childbirth.)

Through our research collaborations, we have published over thirty research articles and book chapters jointly. We have been invited together to speak at national and international meetings. In our research community of national and international reproductive biologists, scientists referred to us as "the Fields brothers." This was years before they realized we were actually brothers.

Michael has retired, and it is sad to look back knowing those are bygone research days. We had been on the top of our research game, and best of all, we were there together.

• • •

I was fortunate to have grown up with three brothers. The other two are Russell Cross and Tim Farrar. Of course, Russell and Tim are not my blood brothers. They are Michael's best friends and have been since grade school. Yet, I will always consider them brothers.

When Michael was old enough to drive, the three of them began including me in many of their adventures. I often wondered if Mom forced Michael into taking me so that he could use her car. If so, no one ever confessed. (Although Tim once said, "We don't mind letting you tag along because you keep your mouth shut afterwards." I will continue my silence about many of the incidents that occurred on those adventures.)

One exploit I can share. During the summer before my brothers' senior year of high school (1961), the Sumter County extension office hired an assistant county agent, Rollin McNutt. In addition to working with the county farmers and ranchers, he was in charge of the county's 4-H program. Having been on the livestock judging team at the University of Florida, it was only natural that he created the first Sumter County 4-H livestock judging team. The four of us were the first members.

Even though we knew absolutely nothing about judging when we joined the team, we won the State Livestock Judging Contest at the Tampa State Fair our first year. I guess you could say Rollin was an excellent coach. One thing is certain: We developed a bond with Rollin that lasted until his death in 2005.

After graduating from high school (1962), Michael and Russell went to the University of Florida and studied animal science. Tim went to Florida State University to study law enforcement. Every year after the football game between the Florida Gators and the Florida State University Seminoles, the winning alumni make a phone call to the losing one or ones. The alumnus of the winning team claims bragging rights (liberally exercised) for another year.

There was a large void in my being when the three of them left for college. Even though it was a painful reminder that my brothers were not around, I remained on the livestock judging

67

team. I did not want to let Rollin down since he was depending on me to mentor new team members.

Two years later, during my senior year of high school (1965), our team again won the state judging contest. This time, I scored first out of about 300 competitors. A month later, the top twenty scorers in the state contest competed in a judging contest at the University of Florida. The top four from that contest represented Florida at The International Livestock Exposition in Chicago, IL. I placed first in that contest also. I was excited, but not because of the personal accolades. Since I was first, Rollin would be the assistant coach for the Florida 4-H team. The University of Florida livestock judging coach, Dr. Don Wakeman, was the head coach. He had been Rollin's coach at the University of Florida, so this had to have been one of those proud moments for both the student and the teacher.

I felt proud to have contributed to the recognition that Rollin received for the judging team's success. He was one of those special people in my journey. Rollin taught me the importance of hard work and never taking the easy road to reach an ultimate goal. He once said, "People do not become successful because they are led by situations. They become successful because they follow a dream."

I have always attempted to follow Rollin's advice to have a plan for where I wanted to go, what I wanted to be, or what I wanted to accomplish.

Now, though, I was at MD Anderson Cancer Center, and circumstances over which I had no control were leading me. I had no plan, since I did not know anything about my leukemia. I was entirely without a vision.

Because of the people I encountered in my life who helped shape my character, I would eventually develop a plan. I would grab my passion for running marathons by the throat and begin a journey down a long road to a dream. I would tell leukemia, *Thank you very much. You are more than welcome to try to keep up with me during this trip.*

• • •

What became of my other two brothers?

Russell received his PhD and moved to Washington, D.C., where he worked with the U.S. Department of Agriculture (USDA). He quickly developed a national reputation for his work ethic, and he was highly sought after by the food industry because of his talents. He worked with the USDA's Food and Safety Inspection Service under Presidents Bush and Clinton; was vice president of IDEXX Labs in Portland, Maine; was the CEO for Future Beef Operations in Parker, Colorado; was vice president of DuPont in Wilmington, Delaware; and was the executive vice president of National Beef in Kansas City, Missouri, to name a handful.

As chairperson of the Animal Science Department at Texas A&M University, he expanded his talents internationally and consults with the U.S. government regarding agricultural trade.

I have Russell to thank for my time at Texas A&M University. You see, Russell also was at Texas A&M University getting his PhD in meat science. He talked the department head into giving me a chance. Therefore, in a way, Russell helped put me on my path to success and that of my second love, Marsha Kay Martin (**Chapter Related Memory: The Chicken Wing.** The story is at the end of the chapter).

Tim graduated from Florida State University with a degree in criminology. In 1967, he joined the U.S. Army and was a Second Lieutenant in the Military Police Battalion at Presidio in

San Francisco. He quickly rose through the ranks: First Lieutenant in the 25th Infantry Division in Vietnam, Commander of a 155 Howitzer Unit, Captain in the U.S. Air Force as a Security Police Squadron Commander, and Lieutenant Colonel and Combat Support Commander.

Later, while in the Army Reserve, Tim worked for The Bureau of Alcohol, Tobacco, and Firearms (ATF). He began as a special agent and was involved in finding and destroying illegal moonshine stills in the backwoods of Mississippi. After Mississippi, Tim's job with ATF took him to Kentucky, where he investigated bombings by members of the Teamsters' Union. He worked his way through the ranks and became Resident Agent in Charge, International Liaison, and lastly Senior Special Agent.

Each year, my three brothers and I get together for a four-day weekend. It is always somewhere different around the country, but the incidents are similar.

For example, in 2015, we met in Key West, Florida. There, we sat by the pool at night with our various favorite alcoholic beverages. As our consumption of drink increased, so did our exaggeration of high school accomplishments, fast cars, and female encounters.

During the day, we walked to tourist attractions such as Ernest Hemingway's home, the historic district, Truman's compound, and the Waldorf Astoria Resort. While playing tourist, we drank from coconuts and discussed current world events and politics.

One afternoon, we went on a sailboat outing. The boat made stops so that those who wanted to could go snorkeling or kayaking among the mangrove trees. We remained onboard and reminisced about the past while enjoying the gentle rocking of the boat, the cool ocean breeze, and the free wine.

With an unlimited supply of wine, the entire boatload of mariners eventually gathered around us, listening to (and laughing at) our tales. We spun yarns about my dissection of cadavers, running marathons, and port-o-let encounters. Michael provided vivid details on pregnancy testing of cows and the collection of bull semen for artificial insemination. They were especially interested in Russell's tenure with the Bush and Clinton administrations and his investigation of the *E. coli* contamination of hamburger meat at Jack-in-the-Box in 1993. I believe they found Tim's accounts of shootouts with Mississippi moonshiners and the investigation of bombings in Kentucky to be most entertaining. The seagulls and pelicans of Key West had never before heard such laughter.

As I lay on my hotel bed in Houston, memories of my three brothers quieted my soul, and with that came sleep.

Chapter Related Memory: The Chicken Wing

Therefore, in a way, Russell helped put me on my path to success and that of my second love.

The year was 1971, and I was working on my master's degree in meat science at Texas A&M University. Marsha Kay Martin was working part-time as a lab assistant in the Meat Science Section while pursuing her undergraduate degree. The section head assigned her to help me collect data for my research project. At first, she went unnoticed. Then later, after getting to know her better, I was head over heels in love.

Marsha invited me over for dinner so that she could introduce me to her parents. Her father looked vaguely like a pit bull and he had a personality to match. When we entered the house, Mr. Martin was watching *Gunsmoke*. As I began to introduce myself, he said, "Quiet. I am watching my favorite TV show. We can talk when it is over."

We had no choice but to sit on the couch and watch *Gunsmoke*. During the show, Marshal Matt Dillon was in a gunfight. As was typical for this TV series, he was slower on the draw but was more accurate with his shot. He always won. As the marshal holstered his gun, Marsha's father finally spoke, "Did you see that? I'm just as tough as that guy."

"Which guy, the one that just got shot?" I responded.

My comment elicited an elbow in my ribs from Marsha.

At dinner, the family passed around a platter of fried chicken. I took half a breast and a wing, and passed the platter to Mr. Martin. As he took the platter from me he said, "You are new here, so let me inform you of the rules. The wings are mine. So keep your damn hands off them."

Later in the meal, Marsha again handed me the platter, and I took a wing. All conversation around the table went silent as everyone, including me, waited for the eruption. Instead of Mr. Martin knocking me off my chair, he laughed aloud. Marsha kicked me under the table.

• • •

The year was 1975. I came home from classes at Texas A&M University and found a letter on my door. Marsha gave some excuse about being too young for a commitment and feeling like there were things she was missing. Like Babs, I still miss her after all these years.

CHAPTER 8

Lost Innocence

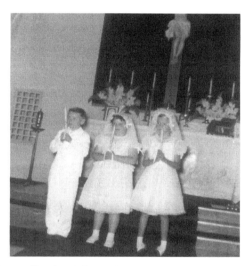

Right to Left: Mary Ellen, Dorothy, and Me
(First Communion, 1955)

I have been driven many times upon my knees
by the overwhelming conviction that I had nowhere else to go.
My own wisdom and that of all about me
seemed insufficient for that day.
Abraham Lincoln[10]

When I awoke from my nap, it was dark outside. I again walked to
Ruby Tuesday for dinner.

While in a dining booth, I thought to myself, *I learned just one thing of significance today: I am only five feet, eight inches tall. I can only assume that the basketball coach exaggerated my height in our basketball lineup so that our team would appear taller. After all these years, I should probably change that information on my driver's license.*

I added "driver's license" to my list of things to do when I returned home. Things like developing an official will and going to confession.

I am not sure if you caught my comment earlier, but I am Catholic. My Catholic identity has been an integral part of my life, and although unsuccessful at times, I have attempted to live a Christian life.

They say that prayer is a way to reach God and to repent. I have always prayed for others, but never for myself. I always felt selfish praying for myself when there were so many other people for whom I cared.

It was not until my leukemia diagnosis that I fully appreciated what it meant to call on God for my own needs. In the coming years, there would be numerous arduous circumstances associated with my leukemia—circumstances that would bring me to my knees and remind me that I was not as tough as I thought I was. I would ask God for help just to make it through the day.

• • •

When I was a young boy, being a Catholic was not always easy. Up until I was ten years old, my family was one of three Catholic families in Bushnell, Florida. With so few of us Catholics around, we stood out and were subject to ridicule at school more than a few times. Friday at lunchtime was the worst. Back then, because of Catholic rules, we could not eat meat on Friday. Mom asked the school to have the cafeteria serve us fish sticks. The noncatholics had some sort of mystery meat.

While looking for a seat at a table in the school cafeteria I would hear, "There's that Catholic with his fish sticks."

"He's too good to eat meat like the rest of us."

"What makes him think he's so special?"

"Hey, fish breath, here's a seat."

• • •

Most people remember precisely where they were when news broke of President Kennedy's assassination, and I am no different. It was 12:30 p.m. Friday, November 22, 1963. I was in the eleventh grade and walking from the high school cafeteria after lunch. The principal announced over the loudspeaker that someone had shot President John F. Kennedy. From that day forward, I would no longer embrace the innocence or security of childhood.

In the schoolyard, several older students were cheering about the news of the shooting. I felt disgusted at their audacity not to even bother trying to hide their excitement. There are times when it is best to keep your mouth shut, something I have never learned to do. (This is a recurring theme in this chapter and, really, in this book.) Since I was a fan of the president, I admonished them for their reaction. They turned on me.

"The only reason you like the president is because he's Catholic," they sneered cruelly.

"No, I like him because I'm Catholic," was my reply.

After the fight, the principal expelled me for three days.

Mom reacted indifferently to the temporary expulsion. After all, she taught me that there are times when you should stand up for your beliefs. Although I believe, she would have preferred that I had done so without fighting.

• • •

When I was old enough for the Sacrament of Confirmation, two nuns drove to Bushnell from Leesburg twice each month to teach catechism classes to my friends, Dorothy and Mary Ellen, and myself. My brother went through Confirmation several years earlier.

To me, these nuns were scary in their black habits with their black-and-white pterodactyl-like headpieces. They expected silence and an unquestioning obedience to their teachings. I was a slow learner in both respects.

Once, the nuns were discussing how caring and loving God was. I raised my hand and reminded them, "On your last visit, you told us that God got so angry with his people that he instructed Moses to build a boat. God then flooded the earth, killing almost everything. The only people or animals that survived were on the boat. Did Moses also take two cockroaches?"

There was no response from the nuns, so I assumed that they were interested in what else I had to say. It never occurred to me that they might have been in shock over my comments.

Consequently, I kept speaking, "And then God destroyed Sinbad and Gonorrhea? He even turned someone's wife into a lot of salt. That doesn't sound very loving."

To the nuns' consternation, my verbal discourse prompted laughter from the other two pupils. Probably because I did not get the story of Noah, Sodom and Gomorrah, or of Lot's wife correct.

Back then, I did not have all the religious facts correct. I confused biblical stories with TV shows.

Early on, I wondered why the nuns carried an eighteen-inch wooden ruler. Because of my errors of biblical events, my bruised knuckles answered my question. I wanted to ask, *What is a cubit?* I refrained from doing so since my knuckles had had enough.

• • •

Later, more Catholics moved into Bushnell. Among them was Dr. Hume. He and his family lived in a large old house that also served as his doctor's office. He donated a back room to the parishioners, who converted it into a chapel. A priest drove over from Leesburg each Sunday to say Mass. Under the priest's training, my brother and I became the first altar boys in Bushnell.

Back then, the priest recited the Mass in Latin. I was only in the sixth grade but had memorized the entire liturgy. I could recite the Kyrie eleison and *et cum spiritu tuo* with as much fervor and devotion as anyone. Of course, I did not have the foggiest idea what any of it meant.

Midnight Mass on Christmas Eve and the Stations of the Cross during Lent were my favorite services. My job as an altar boy was to carry and swing the incense burner. To this day, that smell brings back so many wonderful childhood memories—and an allergy attack.

I remember my first Midnight Mass in Leesburg. The altar boy at that church was enthusiastically swinging the incense burner, and the inside of the Church became enveloped in a fog of incense. My sinuses were hyperactive, and I was sniffling like a bird dog tracking quail. This apparently annoyed the parishioner in the pew in front of us, who turned around and handed me a handkerchief. I accepted his offering in embarrassment since it felt like everyone in the church was watching me.

As our congregation in Bushnell grew, Michael and I trained additional altar boys. Eventually, the parishioners built St. Lawrence Catholic Church, and they purchased an organ. My new responsibility was organist.

The priest told an amazing story at the church's dedication. Sometime during the early third century AD, a man named Lawrence was one of seven deacons (servants) who provided help to the poor and the needy in Rome. At that time, the Romans persecuted the Christians for not paying homage to their pagan gods. Pope Sixtus II and Lawrence were among those who were condemned to death. (Being a youngster, the next part of this story really got my attention.)

The Romans tied Lawrence to the top of an iron grill and slowly roasted him over a fire. Having so much love for God, he did not feel the flames. He told the executioner, "Turn me over—I'm done on this side!" Then, just before he died, he said, "It's cooked enough now."

• • •

Many years ago, I experienced a similar situation. However, the difference was that my faith was not as strong as Lawrence's was, so I felt the pain.

It was 1965, my first semester at Lake Sumter Junior College. Mom was having the Florida room of our home expanded. The new addition had a flat roof. To save Mom money, I helped the builder. My job was to place large chunks of tar in the cooker. I then filled a bucket with the molten tar, carried it up the ladder, and poured it on the roof. The builder and I then smoothed the tar with mops before it solidified.

It was the middle of the summer, and it was hot, especially around the cooker. My clothing consisted of shorts and a pair of loafers in which I had cut the toes out. No socks.

It was getting late, and after working in the heat all day, I became weary. While lifting a bucket of the molten tar onto the roof, the bottom of the bucket caught on the top rung of the ladder and the hot liquid poured out. Looking down, I could not see my left leg and shoe. The tar had created a solidified cast around both. I climbed down the ladder, turned the hose on, and began running water over my blackened cast.

Mom came outside to see why tar was dripping onto the patio and saw what had happened. She called Dr. Hume and rushed me to his office. On my way to the doctor's office, I had two thoughts: *How is the doctor going to remove this tar cast from my leg and this shoe from my foot? Will he be able to do both without peeling all my skin off?* I concluded: *When he attempts this, it is really going to hurt.*

Dr. Hume did not skip a beat when we arrived. He submerged my left lower extremity in its tar cast into a type of soapy solution. He then began to make slices in the tar cast with a scalpel. I was fortunate to have hairy legs. Most of the tar had immediately solidified upon contact with the hair instead of with my skin. After making slices in the tar cast, he went underneath with scissors, cut the hair, and removed the slices. Unfortunately, unlike a Hobbit, my foot was not hairy and had no protection. That skin came off with the tar and shoe.

Dr. Hume confined me to bed for a month. Since my mother was the county health nurse, I was probably better off at home than in a hospital. (Seriously, if you want to get a life-threatening infection, undergo an extended stay in a hospital.)

Mom smeared a thick yellow salve (Butesin Picrate) over my thigh, leg, and foot several times each day to prevent infection and reduce the pain. It worked much better at the former.

The doctor began making periodic visits to our home for the purpose of debridement, an unpleasant process that is common with severe burns. He accomplished this by cutting away the dead tissue on my leg and foot in order to promote the healing process. This procedure likewise removed a source of tissue where bacteria would thrive.

Dr. Hume was amazed at my lack of utterance during both the tar removal and the debridement. Consequently, on one of his visits to remove skin, he commented, "If you don't show any sort of emotion, I am going to stick the point of these scissors in your foot!" I guess God blessed me with a high threshold of pain tolerance.

In the near future, endless needles, bone marrow biopsies, chemotherapy, and running marathons with leukemia would truly test my tolerance for pain and discomfort.

• • •

I will now return to my trip to the MD Anderson Cancer in Houston, Texas. It was January 2008. Back at the hotel after dinner, I went straight to bed. There was no reason to call anyone and discuss what had happened that first day at MD Anderson Cancer Center. Besides, being a private person, I had not yet informed anyone about my leukemia. If I had let people into my new world of leukemia, they would be asking questions, to which, at that time, I had no answers.

While lying in bed, I reflected on how quickly my life had changed. I had been cruising along without a care in the world, preparing to return to the Boston Marathon for a third time. Then, in the blink of an eye, every plan I had for the future seemed to disappear as quickly as if I had hit the "Delete" button on my computer.

Throughout my life, I have encountered people who knew that something was wrong. Yet, they avoided going to a doctor for fear that it would be bad news. I used to think, *How dumb.* I now have a better appreciation for what they were feeling.

In my experience, a diagnosis of cancer was a death knell. In 1933, my mother's youngest sister died from Hodgkin's lymphoma. In 1988, my dad suffered and died because of cancer. I have had friends whose nieces or nephews had leukemia. They spoke of the horrific ordeal these children went through during chemotherapy. They described how devastating it was for the families during the child's hospitalization and then, sometimes, during the funeral.

I remember the first time I had a personal encounter with death. I was sixteen years old. The husband of a woman who worked with and was a close friend of Mom had a home on Lake Panasoffkee, Florida where he took me duck hunting. He was a heavy smoker and developed lung cancer. One weekend, Mom took me to the hospital to visit him. I was warned before going into his room that he had not recognized anyone for several days and that he did not have long to live.

Entering his room, I was shocked at how emaciated he was. As I approached his bed, he opened his eyes, reached out, took my hand, and smiled. He then said my name and died. He just passed away, right there in front of me.

I was overwhelmed with sadness as I stood there holding his hand. He was a friend, and I had just watched him die.

Now, I was dealing with my own diagnosis. My mortality was front and center in my thoughts. This was not a pleasant experience. I needed a potent diversion, something to replace thoughts of dying. Consequently, I focused on memories of the Boston Marathon to get me through that extremely depressing trip to MD Anderson.

(The upcoming chapters will describe my long history with the Boston Marathon.)

CHAPTER 9

Defining Real

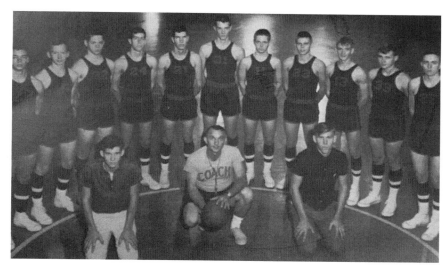

**South Sumter High School Basketball Team
(Second from Right, 1965)**

The starting point of all achievement is desire.
Napoleon Hill[11]

After the Pleasure Island Marathon (1984), it was obvious that my personal library needed more information about running in a race, especially the 26.2-mile mammoth event, the marathon. I purchased a *Runner's World* magazine that contained exactly what I needed: an outline of several marathon-training programs and a list of regional marathons.

New Orleans had a marathon on January 12, 1985—The Great Marathon. I set a goal to finish my second marathon in four hours. Why did I pick four hours? It was faster than my first marathon, and it seemed like a time I could achieve, that is, if I did not stop to take a nap.

When the day of the marathon arrived, I was anxious to test my preparation with one of the marathon-training programs I found in *Runner's World* magazine.

First, a port-o-let stop. I have learned that it makes no difference how many bathroom breaks I take before a marathon; there is always a need for one more. Obviously, this is not unique to me, since the lines in front of the port-o-lets are always long.

Having completed my prerace port-o-let ritual, I found my way to the starting line. Having learned my lesson at the Pleasure Island Marathon, my location was 10 rows behind the front-runners.

On race day, the temperature was going to be in the teens, so I purchased a navy blue cotton sweat suit. Even though I was color coordinated, no amount of Vaseline would have prevented the inner thigh chaffing that I developed that day.

In addition, by mile 6, the front of my sweat suit was solid with ice from water I had spilled while trying to run and drink at the same time. (Unlike my first marathon, I did not pause to drink in the middle of the water stops.)

I had purchased a Timex Ironman thirty-lap watch. I now had a watch with more buttons, and I felt like a real runner. (Key words: *felt like*.)

I completed my second marathon in 3:52, forty-three minutes faster than my first marathon. I placed 360th out of 1,000 runners. I was beginning to enjoy running marathons.

• • •

My third road race was the Causeway Half Marathon, February 17, 1985. The race started at Battleship Park in Mobile, Alabama, home of the battleship *USS Alabama.* (As a kid, I loved building model ships, especially those modeled after ancient and historical vessels: "Old Ironsides" (nickname of the *USS Constitution*), *HMS Bounty*, and the pirate and Viking ships. I enjoyed stringing the ship rigging, making sails, and painting the cannons and miniature sailor figurines. How the pieces all fit together to create such an intricate model entranced me.)

The Causeway Half Marathon course was across Mobile Bay. The Bay is a wildlife sanctuary. So along the course, I saw egrets, gray and white pelicans, an enormous rat, and an alligator crossing the road—definitely not things that you would normally encounter during your typical road race. Later, I learned that the large rat was a nutria—a large rodent that looks like a large rat or a beaver.

The race finished at the armory in a town named Daphne. Drivers transported runners in bright yellow school buses back to the starting line where we had parked our vehicles.

• • •

Riding a school bus has generated numerous fond memories. This is just one of them. I grew up in Bushnell, a small farming community in Central Florida with a population of about 600. There were no traffic lights; there was a caution light at the one (and only) major intersection. The major hangout for high school students was a walk-up-and-order soda shop called Sip & Bite.

My family lived on a small cattle ranch two miles from town. A yellow school bus was my way of getting to and from school and sporting events.

My favorite high school sport coincidentally was the one I was worst at: basketball. How bad was I? As far as I know, the only reason Coach Stewart allowed me on the team was that when you added him and me, on any given day, there were only enough bodies to have a scrimmage game. (Hence, this was why every athlete was required to play in at least two sports, as mentioned previously.)

Two unforgettable events occurred while playing for Coach Stewart. The first was a man-to-man scrimmage. I drew the short straw and had to guard the coach. Each time he attempted a bounce pass to someone on his team, I kicked the ball out of bounds. Coach would glare at me each time this happened. I interpreted his look as a good sign; after all, being the weakest player on the team, I had foiled his attempt. I beamed, proud of my efforts, and could not wait to receive his gesture of respect again.

This scrimmage continued—Coach Stewart attempting a bounce pass and me kicking the ball out of bounds—before he finally broke. He grabbed me by my T-shirt and stuck the basketball in my face. "Kick this ball again, and you are going to eat it!" he growled.

I was stunned. I had obviously mistaken the meaning of his previous glares.

Sure enough, I instinctively kicked his next bounce pass out of bounds. I looked at coach, who menacingly looked back. He then began chasing me around the gym, throwing the basketball at me. Today, coaches probably cannot do that. In fact, Coach Bob Knight could have learned more than a few things from Coach Stewart.

After several missed attempts at trying to hit me with the basketball, Coach Stewart got even angrier. I next witnessed one of the most unforgettable moments in my journey through life, an event that was so incredible that you could never script it in a movie and catch it on film. Coach Stewart dropkicked the basketball straight to the top of the gym. All the players stood there awestruck as the basketball sailed into the upper confines of our old gymnasium. That basketball was like an interceptor missile. It had locked onto a light fixture, one of those large, round, hanging fixtures with a heavy-gauge wire cage to protect the bulb.

It was as if time slowed while everyone stared skyward at the basketball. Then, time sped up with the sound of breaking glass that showered the gym floor. The protective wire cage did not work as designed.

Coach suspended practice, and I remained behind doing sprints back and forth on the basketball court. Running and stopping, running and stopping with every blast of coach's whistle. Thinking back on those memories of high school, my sport coaches were unknowingly preparing me to run a marathon.

The second memory is my most embarrassing and happened in my senior year at our homecoming game. Because a nasty virus was making the rounds, we only had seven players, and there was a good chance I would get to play. If so, I had a chance of lettering. To letter, you had to score at least one point during basketball season. Lettering meant I would be considered a real basketball player (at least, in my mind).

When a second player on our team fouled out of the game, my time had arrived. At least I thought it had. Coach Stewart looked down the bench. He slapped his towel on the floor and said, "Damn, I have no one left to send in."

He finally relented and let me play.

Before I stepped onto the court, he grabbed me by my jersey and got right in my face. (He always seemed to be doing that maneuver with me.) He told me how useless I would be trying to defend our end of the court. Of course, he said this loud enough for everyone in the home bleachers to hear. I could feel my face turning red with embarrassment. Then quietly, he snarled before letting go of my jersey, "Stay at their end of the court when they are trying to score, and wait under their basket."

After the visiting team scored a basket, a player on our team inbounded the ball by throwing it the length of the basketball court. Before I know it, the basketball hit me in the chest, knocking the wind out of me. Coach Stewart failed to tell me that part of the plan. I thought that I was just supposed to stand at the other end of the court–where I was watching our lovely cheerleaders.

Instinctively, I grabbed the ball off the floor and tossed it up. This was excitement at its best; I had finally gotten to play, and now I was actually going to score a basket. I was going to letter.

Not so fast. In front of bleachers full of classmates, I completely missed the backboard, rim and basket. To make things worse, I retrieved the ball before the defenders arrived and took a second shot. This resulted in a second miss.

Out of the corner of my eye, I could see Coach Stewart jumping up and down. He was slapping his towel on the floor, the chairs, and the two players who had failed to clear out of his path. Like everyone in the gym, I could hear him cursing.

I was the topic of ridicule at the homecoming dance after the game.

Nevertheless, I did manage to score a point on a free throw. Later in the game, while dribbling the basketball for a layup, I tripped over my own feet. I fell in front of the defender, and the referee thought the player had tripped me. As I stood at the foul line, the pressure was mounting. I could feel my heart beating. I looked toward the bench—a big mistake. I could see Coach Steward twisting the towel in anticipation. I was shaking so badly that I was afraid the ball would not make it to the basket. It did not.

Everyone in the gym could hear Coach Stewart cursing again. I was afraid to look in his direction, but I could hear the towel hitting unseen objects. I wanted to believe it was because he also wanted me to score a point and letter.

My level of fear had now increased for my second attempt. The gym had gone silent. I thought, *Is it my imagination, or is that the sound of a towel being twisted into a knot?*

Swoosh! I was now a real basketball player; I lettered.

Oh, I almost forgot, we won the game in spite of me.

That was the only time that I played in the two years that I was on the team. Even so, I always looked forward to practice. The more Coach Stewart harassed me, the more I liked him. After all, he was a challenge.

Forty years later, during one of my monthly visits to Mom, I crossed paths with Coach Stewart in the Bushnell Wal-Mart parking lot. After a lengthy visit to catch up on past and current things going on in our lives, I asked, "Coach, why did you get so angry that day at practice when I kept kicking your bounce passes?"

He explained, "I wanted you to use your hands and try to catch the ball. That way, we would have possession."

Gosh. I thought. *Why didn't he just say that back then?*

At least after all these years, I now know the answer.

I was saddened to hear of Coach Stewart's death shortly after our encounter. Of all the high school teachers, he had the biggest impact on my development. He had taught me not to quit in the face of adversity, regardless of how bad things got. Believe me: As a basketball player, I was bad. This amazing basketball coach taught me important skills that I would need to survive hardships, marathons, and now, my battle with cancer. Perhaps this is why these particular memories stand out so much to me, even this long after the fact.

• • •

After that high school digression, let me take you back to the Causeway Half Marathon in February 1985. Had I not ridden that particular school bus after the Causeway Half Marathon, I might never have learned about the Boston Marathon. As it turned out, that bus ride radically changed my life forever.

In the seat in front of me, there was a guy flirting with one of the female runners. He wore a green jacket with a Boston Marathon emblem. That was the first time I met Mike "Mad Dog" Sealy. It was not the last time that I would see him flirting with a female runner at, during, or after a race.

I tapped him on his shoulder. "What is the Boston Marathon, and how can I get one of those jackets?"

He turned around and gave me an odd, incredulous look. "You don't know about the most prestigious marathon in the world?"

"Mad Dog" probably thought that I was an ignoramus. In spite of my ignorance, he continued talking to me. "The Boston Marathon is the only marathon you have to qualify to run. And you will have to qualify in order to get a jacket like this."

He then asked me my age. After I provided him that information, he quoted the time that I would need to finish a marathon in order to qualify. His conversation continued with places and things at the Boston Marathon that absolutely made no sense to me. He spoke about a place called "The Common," a school bus ride to an athletic village in Hopkinton, screaming women at a college called Wellesley, and on and on. He was a walking encyclopedia on the Boston Marathon.

Lastly, he informed me, "You will not be considered a real runner until you qualify for and run Boston." He then went back to his flirtation.

I spent the rest of the bus ride chasing one thought after another. *After just two marathons, my best time is 3:52. I am thirty-eight years old and need to run a 3:10 marathon in order to qualify for Boston. So, all I need to do is shave another forty-two minutes off my previous marathon time. That is doable; after all, my finishing time between my first and second marathons improved by forty-three minutes. I accomplished this in less than ten months of training. In addition, I just ran the Causeway Half Marathon in 1:35. That is half of 3:10. Surely, after another year of training, I will qualify.*

During that bus ride, I set a goal: I would become a real runner. From that day forward, I was a completely different person. The Boston Marathon became as much a part of my being as any part of my physical body. I was possessed. My desire to run the Boston Marathon would never be any further in my daydreaming than the length of a neuron in my brain.

CHAPTER 10

The Team

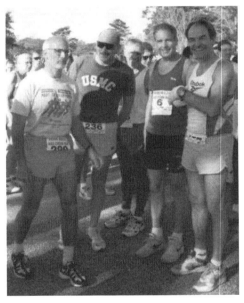

Left to Right: Tom, Mike, Me, Don, Larry (1995)

Don't walk behind me; I may not lead.
Don't walk in front of me; I may not follow.
Just walk beside me and be my friend.

Albert Camus[12]

For the next decade, I diligently followed that professional marathon-training program but never got my time under three hours and thirty minutes. After twenty-three failed attempts, many runners likely would have thrown in the towel. Someone even suggested, "Maybe you just don't have what it takes to qualify. Maybe you should stop trying."

There was no way I was going to stop trying. I had a passion (I hesitate to say "obsession") for the Boston Marathon, and I was not about to give up. After all, I became a real basketball player against all odds. I would become a real runner.

You are probably asking, "What makes the Boston Marathon so much more special than all the other marathons?" For one thing, runners cannot just show up and run the Boston Marathon. First, they have to qualify on a certified marathon course. It is the challenge of qualifying for Boston that really sets it apart and makes it unique. Only 1 percent of runners ever run a marathon, and only 10 percent of those ever qualify to run the Boston Marathon.

The other question you may be asking is, "Why keep using a training program that obviously was not working?" Well, like the high school football equipment, I simply did not know better. I had not yet figured out what I needed to achieve my goal. In the words of *Dirty Harry*, "A man's got to know his limits."

What I had not yet figured out is that, for a middle-of-the-pack runner like me, the training program I was using—with too little mileage and not enough speed work—would not work. It would not allow me to reach my limit.

I was not lacking in desire. I was learning what the problem was by trial and error. I ran alone and did not have the advantage of running with people who knew how to properly train. Yet, as an introvert, I loved the solitude that came with running alone. There was none of the annoying chitchat. In 1991, that all changed when I began running with a bizarre bunch of runners I call "The Team."

Each runner on "The Team" has a nickname. Don "The Stallion" Wright, our fastest runner, was chair of the communications department at the University of South Alabama. Unlike the rest of us, he had a running pedigree. He ran cross-country at Washington State University between 1964 and 1967, and he was the team captain there in 1966 and 1967.

Don got his nickname because, at the time, he was one of the better runners in the southern region. He was like a thoroughbred when he ran. He could dig deep into the pain and find another gear if someone challenged him. He did not like losing and rarely did so.

Don was the more outspoken member of our team. He introduced me to the proper technique for responding to a driver who pulls out and blocks the sidewalk we were running on. He would slap the car as if the driver had hit him. He would then scream, "You [expletive] idiot!" Don loved to use the word *idiot*.

Mike "Mad Dog" Sealy—the same Mike that I met on the bus after the Causeway race—was an ex-marine and an engineer at a chemical plant. He was a good golfer as well (remember this for later). Someone gave Mike his nickname before we met. One rumor was that a rabid "mad" raccoon had bitten him and rabies shots were required (for Mike, not the raccoon). A more credible story is that someone heard him barking at an attractive female runner during a race.

Larry "Cut the Course" Holmes was a professor in the history department at the University of South Alabama. I first met Larry while running around the University of South Alabama's campus. He was running with Mike, who introduced us by saying, "This is Larry Holmes. He's a state champion."

The first words out of Holmes's mouth was, "Don't talk to him. He's not a real runner." Larry was referring to me.

My mind traveled back to 1985 when Mike had told me I would not be a real runner until I had qualified and run the Boston Marathon. I wondered, *Did Larry run the Boston Marathon?* (He had not done so, but not because he could not qualify.)

The Team met each day at noon at the university gym for a ten-mile run. Larry always got to the locker room early, dressed out, and began running before the rest of us.

One day, Don was talking about the cemetery we ran past. Larry asked, "What cemetery?" Eventually, we discovered why Larry did not know about the cemetery. He was cutting the course. He never went past the cemetery. Don hid one of his racing trophies under a bush near the cemetery but did not tell Larry. Don's plan, as conveyed to us, was to present the trophy to Larry if he ever ran that portion of the course. Ten years later, the trophy was still there.

Over the years, it did not matter what course we ran. Larry would start early and then cut more off the course than a barber cuts hair off at military boot camp. Thus, Larry's nickname–"Cut the Course".

Next, there was Tom "Slut Runner" Root, a building contractor and a buyer and seller of real estate. He would run any course a team member wanted to run and as fast as the team wanted to run. Just do not ask him to pick the course or set the pace. Because of this, Larry came up with Tom's nickname.

Lastly, Dave "Politically Correct" Gartman was a professor in the political science department at the University of South Alabama. He was so politically correct that he would try to run off and leave us if anyone started telling jokes. Consequently, everyone told jokes.

Dave quit running with us shortly after I joined the group. A rumor circulated that his wife told him to stop seeing us because we were corrupting him. That rumor was unsubstantiated.

I would be remiss not to include Glenn "The Coach" Sebastian, chair of the geography department at the University of South Alabama. Although Glenn did not run, he served an important role: He was our coach of sorts. He e-mailed us words of encouragement or inspirational poems before each race.

My nickname would come much later (Chapter 26)

• • •

The Team's motto was "Winners finish first. All the rest are losers." Consequently, they were always competing against each other, even in the workouts. You may have noticed that I said "they" and not "we". These guys were fast and I was no competition.

You had to be careful when you attempted to pass Larry. He was so competitive that he would weave, elbow, or cut you off at the corners. He took the motto too seriously. In one particular 5K race, Mike attempted to pass Larry on the inside at a street corner. Following a shove from Larry, Mike ended up on a water station table with cups of water flying everywhere.

Once each week, we went to the track for a workout called "thousands"—1,000 yards. The rules were simple. First, everyone took turns leading a 1,000-yard repeat. Second, we could not pass the leader except in the last 200 yards. That was not a problem for me since I was at least 100 yards behind the last one to cross the finish line.

Tom would hang back each "thousand" and talk the whole time, except for the "thousand" he led. One day, Dave got mad and yelled, "[Expletive] Tom, if you can talk during the workout, you are not running hard enough."

We were all stunned. That was the first time we had heard Dave curse. That also was the last time we heard him curse; he stopped running with us. Maybe his wife was correct; we were corrupting him.

I hated when it was my turn to lead because I was so much slower than everyone was. They would be behind me the first 800 yards, screaming obscenities. "Come on Fields, pick it up! This is supposed to be a track workout. If we had known you were this slow, we would have brought a twenty-four-hour clock to time us." (Of course, this is not the X-rated version that I had to endure.)

• • •

The following event occurred before I joined The Team.

It started with Don belittling Larry, saying, "Every day you start our run early, you then cut the course, and I still beat you back to the gym."

To this Larry responded, "Yes, but I'm not racing. If I were, you would be eating my dust."

Don issued a challenge to Larry to race their ten-mile course. According to the rules, Larry would have a five-minute head start and could run his abbreviated course.

The Coach sat in the back of a pickup truck with a movie camera and filmed the race. Mike drove the truck, and Tom was in the passenger seat. Don, "The Stallion," caught up to Larry with less than three miles to the finish and won. The film continued to show up at team gatherings to remind Larry for years after the fact.

The next story is one that Larry has told and retold so many times that, if it were a paperback novel, the cover would be worn off.

Larry travels to Russia each summer and spends time in the library archives somewhere in Siberia. He writes books on the history of Russian education and politics. Upon returning from Russia one summer, Mike called Larry and said, "I have been running with a really good runner over the summer, and he is going to join us today."

Larry inquired, "Who is this runner?"

Mike responded, "I don't know his name."

Larry cackled before saying, "So, you have been running with this guy all summer, and you don't know his name?"

The runner was Tom, but the story does not end there.

Larry and Mike took Tom on a run over one of their courses through forest trails behind the university. The trails curve around for miles and crisscross each other. It is easy to get lost in those woods. After getting deep into the woods, Mike and Larry sped up. Their plan was to run off and leave Tom. After Mike and Larry completed the workout, considerable time passed but Tom did not appear.

Larry asked Mike, "Do you think we should go back and look for your friend? He might be lost."

Mike responded, "You can go look for him if you want. I'm going home to eat pork chops."

Mike went to dinner and Larry waited at the trailhead for Tom. After about an hour Tom appeared and he was not in a good mood.

The events in the next story happened long before Don or I joined the team. Mobile organized its first marathon (which turned out to be its only one until the First Light Marathon in 2002). Larry had trained hard and was planning on winning. However, at mile 5, Mike was so far ahead of everyone that Larry was now hoping to finish second. Around mile 15, a pickup truck pulled up beside Larry. Mike was in the bed of the pickup truck making obscene gestures, and he even mooned Larry. Later, around mile 23, Mike again pulled up beside Larry. This time he was on a bicycle. No one knows where Mike found a bicycle out on the course, but Larry won the marathon.

That was not the last time Mike pulled such a stunt. Don and Mike were at a ten-mile race. Mike ran the first mile over a minute faster than his mile repeat workouts. As described by Don, "By mile 3, he was so far ahead that I never saw him again. That is until a deputy sheriff pulls up beside me at mile 8 and blows his car horn. It is Mike, and he is giving me the finger."

Again, no one knows where Mike found a sheriff's car. However, long before I knew him, he had been a deputy sheriff. Maybe the car belonged to an officer patrolling the course.

• • •

The guys on The Team lived to run and did not let anything interfere with their passion. I will share a story that justifies the above statement.

We were attending a Friday night baseball game of the Mobile Bay Bears, a Double-A affiliate of the Arizona Diamondbacks. Mike showed up with a woman friend, and he kept looking sheepishly at us during the first two innings. During the third inning, he said, "I have an announcement." He then held up the woman's hand to show us her ring.

We were stunned since we did not know that he was dating anyone.

Later during the baseball game, Mike went for popcorn. We were finally able to have a discussion with his latest love. After much grilling (well, friendly conversation), she informed us, "You guys are too worldly, and Mike spends entirely too much time with you. In fact, he spends too much time playing golf and running. I am going to change all that."

This prompted an outpouring of, "Ha, Ha, Ha. Yeah, right. Good luck with that." Our parting comment to her was, "You do not know Mike very well, do you?"

Mike showed up on Monday for our ten-mile run with a new gold wristwatch, for which he had traded the engagement ring. I guess he was not going to cut back on his running or his golfing.

• • •

I never beat any of The Team members in a workout or a race. Yet, they helped me take my running to a new level, my limit. After all, Don, Mike, and Larry had run marathons in under three hours: Don (2:40), Mike (2:47), and Larry (2:54).

From The Team, I learned the benefit of running long miles faster than race pace, doing speed workouts, and running road races. These all helped me develop the speed and endurance that I needed to qualify for the Boston Marathon.

Lastly, I learned about that sink in the port-o-lets. Don informed me, "You idiot, that isn't a sink; it's a men's urinal."

CHAPTER 11
Finally

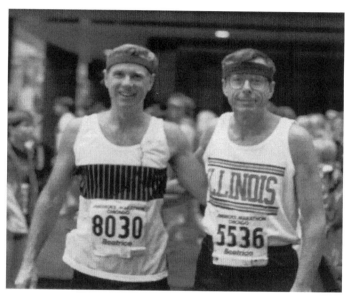

Right to Left: Dave Sherwood and me (Chicago Marathon, 1986)

"Somewhere over the rainbow, skies are blue,
and the dreams that you dare to dream really do come true."
E. Y. Harburg[13]

Before I continue with my story of the Boston Marathon, I need to introduce the fourth love in my life, Leslie.

The year was 1983, long before I joined The Team, when I had another one of those chance encounters that would change my life. For some unknown reason, I stopped running on the roads in the afternoon and began running on the university track. During my prerun stretching, I saw a very beautiful woman running laps on the track. She had the sexiest legs and jet-black hair put up in a cute ponytail that appeared to wave at me with every step she took. I was hypnotized.

I immediately fell in love with her. Yet, it took me two months to build up enough courage to speak to her. When I finally spoke to her, my first words were "Hi" while running past her on the track. Obviously, my technique for impressing women had not improved.

Afterwards my thought was, *You blew that, you dummy*. Nevertheless, like attempting to qualify for the Boston Marathon, I was persistent. I continued to say "Hi" each day when I saw her at the track. My efforts finally paid dividends, and after five years (November 1988), she agreed to marry me.

Leslie brought incredible happiness into my world, and she would play a major role in bringing my biggest dream to life.

• • •

The date was September 1, 1995, seven years after Leslie and I had married. I boarded a train in a suburb outside of Chicago with my good friend and research collaborator, Dave Sherwood. Dave was a professor at the University of Illinois at Urbana-Champaign. We had published several scientific papers and book chapters together on the hormone relaxin and its role in reproduction.

Now, we were on a train to the starting line of the Lake County Marathon, Zion, IL. We would be attempting to qualify for the 1996 Boston Marathon, the marathon's 100th anniversary.

Runners on the train were chatting among themselves. They were discussing previous marathons and the number of marathons they had run, the training programs they used, and the pre-marathon carbs they ate. They were an enthusiastic group, and the decibel level of the dialogue increased precipitously during the first two-thirds of the train ride. Then, as we got closer to the starting area, the noise level decreased. I assumed the runners were beginning to concentrate on the race, something I had been doing since stepping onto the train.

I had been sitting quietly and focusing on my ten-year dream: qualifying for the Boston Marathon. At my age (48), my required qualifying time was 3:25—ten minutes faster than I had run any of my previous marathons.

• • •

The Team had helped me tailor a marathon-training program to reach the height of my running ability.

I continued doing the ten-mile runs with The Team four afternoons a week. Then, on the weekends, I ran a long run of fifteen to twenty-four miles. Wednesday was for speed workouts that I did alone. The speed workouts began with six quarter-mile repeats. I ran these at a pace one minute-per-mile faster than that required to qualify for the Boston Marathon. (I needed to run a 7:50 pace in order to qualify.)

I added two quarter-mile repeats each week until I reached twenty repeats. Next, I began doing half-mile repeats, starting with four at the same pace as the quarter-mile repeats. Again, I added two each week until I reached ten repeats. Last were one-mile repeats at the same pace. I started with five and added two each week until I reached thirteen repeats. I rested two minutes between each repeat. Once I began running the mile repeats, I ran the long runs on alternate weekends. I ran my long runs under the qualifying pace.

• • •

As I sat with my thoughts on the train to the marathon start, I briefly questioned whether my personalized training program had adequately prepared me. After all, I had failed in twenty-three previous attempts. I shook my head to dislodge those thoughts; this was not the time for negative thinking. Instead, I turned my focus to the hard work and positive moments in my training. I recalled the times I had wanted to quit with only one repeat left to run, but I had not quit. I recalled my time trials. The first was fifteen miles at the qualifying pace. Two weekends later, I ran eighteen miles at the qualifying pace. In two more weekends, I failed to hit my target on the twenty-mile time trial. I felt anxious about that shortcoming and feared it would leave a negative emotion in the upcoming race. Consequently, I got up the next morning and ran the twenty miles again, successfully reaching my pace goal.

On the train, I kept reminding myself, *I have properly trained, and I have the necessary desire to achieve this goal. Today I will be another step closer to becoming a real runner.*

This was not simply a yearning of the moment. It was an aspiration of the heart, something I had carried inside me for a decade. Yet, somehow, this attempt seemed more important. Not only was it for qualifying to run in the 100th Boston Marathon, but also I felt that Dave and my family were counting on me doing so. Our families were going to travel together to share in this Boston celebration.

Consequently, I was no longer doing this just for me. Failing was not an option.

I was aroused from my slumber by three short blasts from the train whistle signaling that we were stopping.

While everyone exited the train and headed to the port-o-lets, I used the vacant bathroom in our rail car. I made it to the starting line just in time for the National Anthem. As I stood at attention, I told myself, *I can do this. I will do this!*

At the beginning of the race, it started to rain. I love running in the rain, and God had provided me with a magic elixir. I was in my comfort zone, and I felt good. I felt confident.

The gun fired, and I was off—off to a date with the Boston Marathon.

Even though Dave was older, by mile 7 he was well ahead of me and out of sight. That did not matter. The only thing of importance was what I did. I had to run my own race and not pay attention to what others around me were doing.

Around mile 17, a runner pulled up beside me and inquired, "What pace are you running? You have been steady."

"I have been keeping it between 7:35 and 7:40 each mile." I responded. "I am trying to qualify for Boston."

"What time do you need to qualify?" He asked.

"Three hours and twenty-five minutes."

He was my age and attempting to qualify for Boston as well.

"So, how are we doing?" He questioned.

I checked my Timex Ironman watch and responded, "We are doing great. We have around a three-minute cushion with less than nine miles to go. Stay with me, and we will carry each other to Boston."

Thankfully, that was his last question. I did not need to be wasting energy with a lengthy conversation. I needed to focus on my running form and listening to my body.

I had never felt so good while running a marathon, and there was no doubt in my mind that I would qualify for Boston.

Until this point, the course had been flat. Shortly after my feel-good moment, I saw the first of many long hills that would see me all the way to the finish. I briefly panicked: *Hills were not part of my training program.* I could not do anything about that now. I had to continue pushing and to trust in my training. I took a deep breath as I mentally prepared to conquer the first hill.

At mile 23, I started up another one of those long, steep hills. By now the muscles of my calves and thighs burned. I had long ago depleted my glycogen reserves, and the Snickers I had just eaten provided no relief. I wanted to stop and join the long stream of runners who were walking up that hill. However, I kept pushing, and pushing, and pushing. I did not think I would ever reach the top. At the summit, I looked back and saw my new friend among those walking up. I was now on my own.

I checked my watch to evaluate my pace in the previous mile. My heart stopped; the stupid thing had a blank screen. The battery had given out. So much for that old saying, "Timex: It takes a licking and keeps on ticking."

I was no longer able to check my pace, but after those hills, I knew it was going to be close. I just did not know how close. There was no reason to conserve any remaining energy, so I ran as hard as I could. My dream was just around the next corner.

Near the finish, I made a sharp right-hand turn. The finish line was now in sight—only fifty yards away. I could see the clock. I was devastated; the red numbers were 3:25:10. I ran under the banner at 3:25:23. I had missed qualifying by twenty-three seconds.

We went to a celebratory dinner that evening for Dave, who had qualified. Everyone's enthusiasm seemed a bit dampened because of my failure to qualify, and I felt badly about spoiling this important moment for Dave. I had also let my family down, since they had been excited about the possibility of going to Boston.

I was distraught for weeks afterwards and kept thinking, *If only I had not made that one port-o-let stop.*

For the next four weeks, Leslie encouraged me to contact the Boston Athletic Association (BAA). She kept saying, "Maybe the twenty-three seconds don't matter." Just like whenever she would insist that I check the road map or ask for directions after getting us lost on a trip, I did not listen. I felt I could get us back on course by looking at the sun or stars. I could not.

They say that men are better at reading a road map than women, but that men get lost more often. I guess it does not matter if men read maps better if we do not actually read them.

Eventually, I listened to Leslie and went to the BAA website. Wow, was I thrilled that I did. To my great joy, runners had to the fifty-ninth second to qualify. Of course, this is no longer true, and you cannot squeak in anymore. However, this was 1995, and I had qualified for the 100th anniversary of the most prestigious marathon in the world.

After ten years and twenty-three failed attempts to qualify, I was finally going to the Boston Marathon. Just like in the song, *Over the Rainbow,* dreams do come true.

CHAPTER 12

My First Boston Marathon

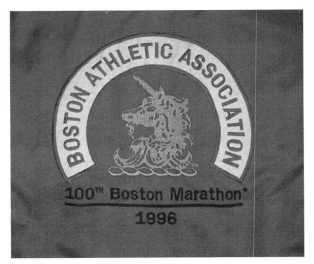

The Official Boston Marathon Jacket (1996)

Dreams are journeys that take one far from familiar shores,
strengthening the heart, empowering the soul.
Pamela Jane Barclay ("Pam") Brown[14]

In April 1996, Leslie, my two stepdaughters Melissa and Courtney, and I flew to Boston. We joined Dave and his wife, Julie, and we stayed at a bed-and-breakfast in Cambridge, Massachusetts.

The day after arriving, Leslie, the girls, and I took the subway into Boston. Being fans of the TV sitcom *Cheers*, we had lunch at the bar and grill for which the show was named. Afterwards, we went sightseeing on the Freedom Trail. Our hike began at Boston Common, which is the oldest city park in the country. I guess people called it "Common" because of its widespread use during America's history. Bostonians used the Common for cattle grazing, town meetings, and public hangings. Prior to the American Revolution, the British troops camped at the site. In April 1775, the British marched from the Common to face colonial resistance at Lexington and Concord.

The park seems to have played a vital part in many illustrious moments of our nation's history. The Common would become a part of my own history. This is where I would depart for Hopkinton, the start of the Boston Marathon.

Next, we visited the Old South Meeting House, where on December 16, 1773, colonists gathered for the Boston Tea Party. The trail continued to the Old State House, site of the reading of the Declaration of Independence on July 18, 1776.

We then walked past Paul Revere's house and the Old North Church. The church became historical on the evening of April 18, 1775 when two lanterns signaled the British were traveling to Lexington and Concord by sea and not land. (Actually, they crossed the Charles River.)

We crossed the Charles Town Bridge to the harbor and boarded the *USS Constitution*. My memory went back some forty years when I had built a model of this ship. Lastly, we toured Bunker Hill, site of a battle during the colonists' siege of British-held Boston on June 17, 1775.

On the day before the marathon, we went to the Marathon Expo. As I stepped inside the convention hall, my memory flashed back to when I first learned about the Boston Marathon in February 1985, a full eleven years previously. I recalled that school bus ride with Mike "Mad Dog" Sealy, interrupting his flirtation to tell me about the Boston Marathon. Now, at the Expo, I was interested in one item only. It was something I had been dreaming about since that bus ride in 1985. I purchased an official Boston Marathon jacket.

Part of what had been an eleven-year quest was now satisfied.

The Boston Marathon occurs on the third Monday in April, Patriots' Day in Massachusetts and Maine. This civic holiday commemorates the first battles of the Revolutionary War fought on April 19, 1775, at Lexington and Concord.

On the morning of Patriots' Day, Dave and I boarded the subway in Cambridge and exited at Boston Common. Here, we joined the tens of thousands of runners already present. We boarded one of the several hundred school buses transporting runners to the marathon's starting area in Hopkinton, Massachusetts.

Around 7 a.m., like the British troops in April 1775 on their way to Lexington and Concord, we departed the Boston Common. However, we were off to a different destination and a different sort of battle.

During the bus ride, I absorbed everything that was happening as I reflected on my eleven years getting to this location. My mind was like a camera, constantly taking photos for future memories of this day.

We stepped off the bus at the Hopkinton High School around 8 a.m. and walked to the athlete village behind the school. The temperature was in the 30s, and it was raining. At the athletic village, the only area left for seating was a large dirt pit. The walls of this crater were about twelve feet high. With the heavy rain, the crater was nothing more than several acres of mud.

Proper positioning in this crater was essential. Along the rim were a hundred or more port-o-lets. In addition, along the rim was a long trough that served as an outdoor latrine for the men. Connections between the individual sections of the trough were not sealed, and urine was leaking down the rim into the pit. Runners at the bottom of the rim were oblivious that something other than raindrops was falling on their heads.

Dave and I entered this basin far from the latrine, sloshed through the mud far out into the center, and spread leaf bags that we had thought to bring with us. There, we sat in the rain and ate soggy bagels while waiting to be called to the race start.

The number on the Boston Marathon race bib reflects your rank according to your qualifying time. At 10:45 a.m., they began calling runners by blocks of numbers to their respective starting corrals. On the way to the start were the school buses that transported us to Hopkinton. In the windows were sheets of paper with series of numbers corresponding to bib numbers. We threw our bags with extra gear through the appropriate window and retrieved them at the finish line.

We made our way through the throngs of runners to our appropriate corral. There, we stood for at least thirty minutes before the race began.

It appeared to me that there were 100,000 people in Hopkinton, with 40,000 runners and spectators included. The exhilaration of being at the Boston Marathon heightened my senses. Even with the less than favorable weather conditions, spectators were on most of the rooftops watching and cheering the runners. The smell of grilled chicken, hamburgers, sausage, and steaks permeated the air. I could hear the Boston Red Sox baseball game playing on radios. The noise was deafening, but it was nothing compared to what I would hear later.

This was a spectacular beginning of an incredible race to Copley Square in downtown Boston.

Don "The Stallion" had warned me: "There won't be any port-o-lets at the corrals so take a plastic bottle. Then, if you need to pee, place the bottle in your running shorts and pee unnoticed." I brought an old centrifuge bottle that was no longer suitable for lab use. As it turned out, Don's advice was excellent.

Typical for Don, he suggested that I throw the bottle to someone in the crowd when the race began. I decided against that advice and found a trash bin along the route for proper disposal.

At noon, a gun sounded the beginning of the race. It had been a long road, but I was realizing a dream that I had held in my heart for 11 years. I was running in the Boston Marathon.

From start to finish, the course drops nearly 400 feet in elevation, achieved with sharp ascents and descents along the way. As far as I could see, there was a wall of runners filling the width of the road. They were going up and down hills. There were places where I could see two hills that runners were cresting. The scene looked like a giant multicolored serpent slithering across the landscape. It was a most spectacular sight.

There are numerous iconic sites along the route. These include the train station in Framingham (mile 5) and the First Congregational Church with its clock tower in Natick (mile 10). Two other iconic places along the course produced extra special memories. Around mile 11, I heard an unusual sound above that of the spectators and runners. With each quarter mile, the sound grew louder until the source of the noise became obvious. Near mile 13, behind metal parade barricades, thousands of women from Wellesley College were screaming as if they were auditioning for a part in the movie *Friday the 13th*. Runners refer to this spot on the course as "the scream tunnel."

Don had advised me to move to the far right side of the road around mile 12, and I did so even though he never explained why. Again, Don's advice was sound: The right side of the road was where all the beautiful Wellesley women lined the racecourse. They certainly were an amorous horde of fillies. I was pinched, squeezed, kissed, and fondled as if I were a piece of fruit in the farmer's market. I felt like these women were testing me for ripeness. By the time I made it through that gauntlet, I was ready for picking. I am still uncertain whether the barricades were there to protect the runners or the Wellesley girls.

I left the scream tunnel with such an adrenaline rush that I surged on the downhill that followed. I paid a price for this folly. In another two miles was the beginning of the Newton hills.

The second memorable place was around mile 18 when I heard a second unusual sound. It sounded like distant thunder, and it grew louder with every step. Reaching mile 20, I was at the bottom of Heartbreak Hill and looking up. This was the last of the four Newton Hills. At the top of the hill was the source of the thunder. There were numerous large drums. Drummers were beating out a cadence for runners climbing to the top of Heartbreak Hill. For many runners, the drumbeat was not sufficient to keep them running all the way to the top. However, thousands of spectators lined the road and mercilessly jeered any runner who stopped to walk. Those runners were soon charging up the hill, and the crowd responded with cheers.

They named this stretch of the course "Heartbreak Hill" in 1936. It was on this hill that the defending champion John A. "Johnny" Kelley overtook Ellison "Tarzan" Brown. Johnny gave Tarzan a consoling pat on the shoulder as he passed. Tarzan apparently thought this gesture was demeaning. He found the strength to catch Kelley and win the race. The newspaper printed, "Breaking Kelley's heart."

Coolidge Corner is located between miles 23 and 24. This is a neighborhood of Brookline, Massachusetts. People named this neighborhood after the Coolidge brothers' general store that opened there in 1857. Here, the spectators lining the road had swelled to fifteen deep. This was nothing, however, compared to what would follow.

Long before I could see them, I heard the 35,000-plus Red Sox fans. They had poured out of Fenway Park at the end of the baseball game to join the race spectators. The baseball game begins early on Patriots' Day so that it ends before the completion of the marathon.

The Boston Globe later estimated that 300,000 spectators had lined the course over the final two miles, which was amazing considering the weather. This is something you just have to experience in person. Words cannot properly describe the sights and sounds of that unbelievable spectacle of humanity.

When I was one mile from the finish, the large CITGO sign was on my left. Shortly after that, I turned right on Hereford Street and then left onto Boylston Street. The finish line was now in sight. The sound was deafening in that last quarter mile. It resonated through my chest such that my heart felt like it was going into fibrillation. After all these years, I can still close my eyes and hear those cheers of 1996.

The sensation I felt when I stepped across the Boston Marathon finish line I had felt before. It was the amazingly wonderful feeling I experienced each evening I returned home from work and saw Leslie.

My exhilaration when I reached the finish line was short lived. Although the rain had stopped, the temperature had dropped below freezing. The buses with the gear bags were what seemed like a mile away to my exhausted legs, even though they were not really that far. I eventually made my way through the mass of humanity and retrieved my bag. Next, there was a line to have the timing chip removed from my shoe.

After that, a volunteer presented me with a Boston Marathon Finisher's Medal. It had been a long journey, but the final chapter of my dream had come true. After all those years and all those failed attempts at qualifying, I had finally run the Boston Marathon.

According to Mike "Mad Dog," I was now a real runner.

• • •

I was thankful for the shiny polyethylene foil blanket they gave us as we crossed the finish line. I was wet and cold as I searched unsuccessfully for Leslie and the girls in the family gathering area.

I entered a tavern, a place to get warm and formulate a plan. I approached the owner, asking, "May I use your phone to place a local call?"

He handed me the receiver and then inquired, "So, you finished the marathon? It was pretty raw out there, wasn't it?"

"Yes, but it was well worth the effort," I responded as I dialed. "I have waited eleven years for this. Now, I am trying to locate my family. I think they have gone back to the place where we are staying." Fortunately, I had carried a card with the phone number of the B&B and placed the call. On the other end of the phone was the owner of the B&B. "Hello?" she said.

"Hi, this is Phillip Fields. Is my wife there?"

"Yes. She and the girls are in the parlor by the fireplace."

"Please tell them I finished and will see them shortly."

I tried not to be angry about them not waiting for me at the finish line. After all, this was something that was extremely important to me, something I had waited a very long time to accomplish. Then I realized the critical word was *me*. I also recalled that if it had not been for Leslie's insistence that I check with the BAA about the twenty-three seconds, I would not be here. Therefore, I could not blame them for not waiting in the miserable rain and cold. Yet, they had left me without any money for the subway.

I explained my dilemma to the tavern owner, and he gave me the necessary money. He also gave me a cup of hot coffee, which helped to warm my insides. I have regretted not returning the next day and repaying him. I should carry a $10 bill in my running shorts pocket for such occasions, but I never seem to remember to do so. (I recall that Dad always carried a $100 bill in his wallet. My brother and I warned him that one day someone would rob him. He responded, "Yes, but it is better to have a happy thief than an angry one.")

Nearly two hours after crossing the finish line, I was back in Cambridge soaking in a tub of hot water and reveling in the events of the day. Not even stranded by my family at Copley Square could dampen my euphoria of having finally run the Boston Marathon.

CHAPTER 13
Counting Marathons

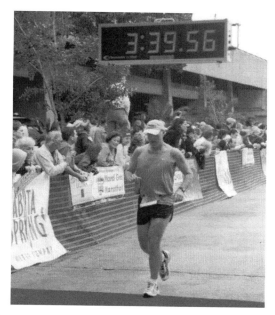

Mardi Gras Marathon, New Orleans (2003)

Seize the moment.
Remember all those women on the 'Titanic'
who waved off the dessert cart.
Erma Bombeck[15]

When I last spoke about my trip to the MD Anderson Cancer Center
(January 2008), it was the end of day 1. I had just returned to my

hotel after dinner at Ruby Tuesday and had gone to bed. As I lay in bed, I reflected on how quickly my life had changed. I recalled my conversations with doctors and nurses about running marathons. In some misguided way, I thought or hoped that if I shared my passion, maybe my prognosis would be better. Upon learning that I ran marathons, they would ask, "How many marathons have you run?"

My response was always the same: "I don't know—I have not kept a count." They all seemed dumbfounded by my response. "You mean, you have been running marathons since 1984 and you haven't counted them?" they would ask, unbelieving.

I tried not to sound arrogant as I explained, "For me, a marathon is just another race. Other than the challenge of the distance itself, it is no different from a 5K or a 10K race. As far as I am concerned, the only marathons worth counting are the Boston Marathon and the ones I qualified to get there. The others are nothing more than failures along my road to Boston."

Now I wondered, *How many marathons have I run?* Giving up on sleep, I got out of bed, turned on my laptop, and began typing notes about past marathons—everything I could remember. When I returned home, I searched through boxes for medals, race certificates, race bibs, or race booklets with results. Even as I did all this, I did not know why. Maybe it was just curiosity. The thought to write all this down in a book would not occur to me for five more years. My motivations for those initial notes were and are a mystery.

The following is a roster of what I learned from my investigation. I have already described my first two marathons: the Pleasure Island Marathon (August 1984) and the Great Marathon in New Orleans (January 1985). New Orleans also had the Mardi Gras Marathon (now called the Rock 'n' Roll New Orleans

Marathon). Although I ran the Mardi Gras Marathon each year between 1985 and 1996, I found only ten finisher medals or racing bibs. That makes twelve marathons.

Having run so many marathons in New Orleans, I would be remiss to pass quickly over the city without commenting on a few sightseeing pleasures. If you visit there, go to the famous Café du Monde in the morning and treat yourself to chicory-flavored coffee and beignets. The Café is located at the edge of Jackson Square. For lunch, enjoy a wonderful Sicilian sandwich called the "Muffuletta." Ride the streetcar that runs down the center of St. Charles Street. Gorgeous old mansions line either side of the road, and they are a magnificent sight. The best time to visit is around Christmas when the residents have exquisitely decorated their homes.

A travel guide lists New Orleans as the most haunted city in the United States. There are twenty-five named ghosts at the Pontchartrain Hotel. Fortunately, the only spirit that I encountered while dining there was the wine.

I do not go to New Orleans without making a dinner reservation at Commander's Palace. My meal is usually the same: An outstanding gin martini, a cup of excellent turtle soup, and pecan-crusted grouper. For dessert, I get a Creole bread pudding soufflé topped with a Bourbon cream sauce that literally melts in your mouth.

If you want to go, make a reservation well in advance and request the garden room. A waiter will take you on a tour through the kitchen and then upstairs to your table. While dining, you can look through the large glass windows out onto a courtyard with sprawling live oak trees that are so emblematic of the South.

Marathon number 13 was in Honolulu, Hawaii, on December 8, 1985. In addition to the heat, I vividly remember the long water stops. They consisted of separate tables for water, a sports drink, and a soft drink. There were three of these setups at each water stop. At the end of each water stop, there were tubs with sponges soaking in ice water. By the time I reached a water stop, the tubs had a strong smell to them—several thousand BenGay-covered runners had inadvertently tossed their sponges back into the tubs. You do not want to grab one and squeeze it over the top of your head. If so, you will spend time going back to a water stop to flush the solution out of your eyes.

Although I finished the Honolulu Marathon with a respectable time of 3:38, I was disappointed. It was not the 3:10 I needed to qualify for the Boston Marathon.

The Chicago Marathon was number 14. In 1986, Dave Sherwood invited me to the University of Illinois in Urbana-Champaign to present a seminar to the reproductive biology department. The invitation was actually an excuse for us to travel to Chicago for the marathon.

Back then, the Chicago Marathon course went by all the famous ballparks. There was Comiskey Park, home of the Chicago White Sox; Wrigley Field, home of the Chicago Cubs; and Soldier Field, home of the Chicago Bears.

Unlike New York, Chicago does not have boroughs; instead, there are various ethnic neighborhoods, and we ran through all of them. During the marathon, there were belly dancers in the Greek neighborhood and mariachi music in the Mexican neighborhood. In the Polish neighborhood, there was folk costume and the smell of delicious grilled sausage. Firecrackers and Dragon dancers greeted us as we ran through Chinatown. My favorite area was Little Italy with the smell of fresh pizza.

The act of running a marathon awakens all of my senses. The event provides memorable sights, sounds, and smells (and afterwards tasting).

The Blue Angel Marathon in Pensacola, Florida, began and finished on the Air Force base. I ran this marathon each year between 1986 and 1996, but I found only eight medals, so I will only count eight. That brings the official tally to twenty-two marathons.

In 1994, I returned to Honolulu for a four-month research sabbatical at the University of Hawaii. Toward the end of my sabbatical, I went over to the Big Island and ran the Kilauea Volcano Marathon. That makes twenty-three. (I will have more to say about that marathon in Chapter 16: "My Hardest Marathon.")

There was a return visit to Illinois in 1995 for the Lake County Marathon, where I qualified for the 1996 Boston Marathon. I am now up to twenty-four marathons. The memories have always been more meaningful to me than the number.

Revisiting memories of these marathons makes me think about all those runners who have completed 300, 500, 1,000 and even 2,000 marathons. Each time I hear those numbers, I wonder, *At what age did they start running marathons? Are they independently wealthy? How do they have that much vacation time? Did they make a commitment at their first marathon to keep count?* It never occurred to me to keep track of my marathons.

The 100th Boston Marathon in 1996 was number 25, and it was my last marathon until 2003. Leslie was doing triathlons and she had been trying to get me to do them with her. Having accomplished my goal of running the Boston Marathon, I started joining her for these events.

Then, during a daily run with "The Team" in June 2002, I suggested that we qualify for the 2004 Boston Marathon. Only Don and Mike were interested. Both had run Boston before, and they understood how special this marathon is.

Our plan was to use the First Light Marathon in Mobile, Alabama (December 2002) to qualify. At mile 15, I developed cramps in my calf muscles, could barely walk, and dropped out. Mike went out too fast and blew up by mile 20. Don was the only one of the three of us who qualified that day.

Mike and I turned to Plan B, the New Orleans Mardi Gras Marathon two months later (February 2003). At mile 20, I heard a sound like a twig snapping. I was not sure what it was until I felt a pain in the bottom of my foot. I knew that if I stopped, the pain would not allow me to start running again. I prayed the last six miles to take my mind off the excruciating pain and ran as hard as my foot allowed. God listened, and I qualified for Boston with a time of 3:40. At fifty-six years old, I needed a time of 3:45 to qualify. Mike also qualified, so the three of us were returning to Boston.

Back home, the orthopedic surgeon said I had developed a long calcium spur in my plantar fascia, likely due to numerous bouts of plantar fasciitis over the years. The spur had fractured during the marathon.

Okay, so, now how many marathons have I run—twenty-six? Is anyone keeping count? Does anyone care? Prior to 2009, I didn't. The number was not important to me. I am repeating myself, but it is true. Back then, marathons were only a means to an end: qualifying for the Boston Marathon.

However, in 2009, tracking my marathons would take on a completely new sense of urgency. With my new companion, leukemia, not only the number of marathons became important, but also the timeframe in which I ran them.

CHAPTER 14
The Power of a Friendly Hello

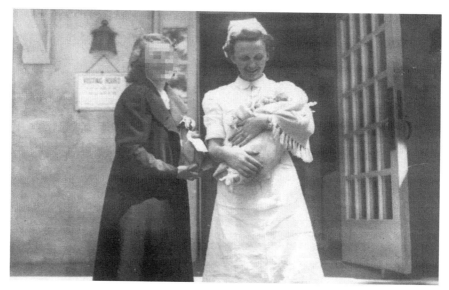

**Mom (right) at the Front Entrance
to the Sumter County Health Department (1945)**

*Instead of asking for God's blessing,
ask how you can be a blessing to others.*
Dr. Kelvin Elko[16]

I was either dating or married to Leslie during all those twenty-six marathons. I have so many great memories of running and of a beautiful woman by my side through it all. One memory in particular occurred during the Honolulu Marathon trip in 1985. After running the marathon, Leslie and I traveled to the island of Maui and stayed at the Sheraton Maui Resort, right on the beach. One evening, while enjoying the view of a full moon over the Pacific Ocean, I gave Leslie a ring and asked her to marry me. Leslie was the most special of my loves. This is probably because I was with her the longest: twenty-one years.

I returned to this same Maui resort hotel in 2008. My brother and I were attending the Fifth International Conference on Relaxin and Related Peptides. That was three years after Leslie and I had divorced and three months after my trip to MD Anderson Cancer Center.

Something sad occurred during that 2008 trip to Maui. My cat Speedi died in her sleep at the vet's office while I was in Maui. She was nineteen years old. I have many fond memories of her. After the divorce, I moved to an apartment complex close to the University of South Alabama, where I worked. Each day when I got home from work, Speedi would meet me at the front door and go out. She would dart across the parking lot at the apartment complex and head straight for the swimming pool. Halfway across the parking lot, she would stop and look back. If I were not following her, she would come back and wait at my feet until I did so. At the pool, I would stretch out on a lounge chair. After Speedi drank from the pool, she would curl up in my lap. As the sun was setting, we would watch the pastel-colored sky. We would continue our vigil by viewing the moon and billions of stars lighting the night.

I am so thankful that I took time out of a seemingly busy schedule to have shared those special moments with Speedi. That is how I remember her.

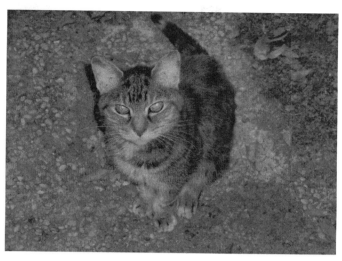

Speedi, My Companion for Nineteen Years (2008)

It seems like the older I get, the harder it is to cope with loss: of friends, of those I love, and even a cat. Although I am in my seventies, I do not seem to be able to manage bereavement well.

Dr. Colin Murray Parkes writes: "The pain of grief is just as much a part of life as the joy of love: it is perhaps the price we pay for love, the cost of commitment. To ignore this fact, or to pretend that it is not so, is to put on emotional blinders. This leaves us unprepared for the losses that will inevitably occur in our own lives, and unprepared to help others cope with losses in theirs."[17]

Also, eloquently written, is this in Ecclesiastes 3:1–8 (King James Version): "To everything there is a season, and a time for every purpose under the heaven: A time to be born and a time to die. …"

Throughout my life, I have asked myself the following question: "Do I live autonomously or belonging to a woman I love?" If I live autonomously, I live by my own set of rules and do what is best for me. Importantly, I do not have to deal with loss. On the other hand, if I live belonging to a woman I love I live by her rules. Everything I accomplish or attempt to accomplish, I do to please her.

Now, as a cancer statistic, I prefer being alone and I do not want pity. I certainly do not want to impose on someone whom I love to take care of me as I deal with a major health issue. I have been fortunate to enjoy four loves; yet, I have also had four losses to cope with.

I was listening to the radio station K-LOVE and a song by For King and Country entitled The Proof of Your Love uses a passage from 1 Corinthians 13:3-7 (The Message), "No matter what I say, no matter what I believe, no matter what I do / if I haven't loved I am bankrupt." I consider myself wealthy.

• • •

The phone in my hotel room rang, interrupting my typing of the information I was compiling about the marathons I had run. It was the wakeup call from the front desk of the hotel that I had requested. Surprised, I looked at the time. I had worked through the night without sleeping.

There were only half as many "Wizard seekers" on the shuttle bus that second morning. Maybe some had already received their bad news and returned home—after spending only one day at MD Anderson Cancer Center, my thoughts had become cynical. I thought, *Surely no one comes to MD Anderson Cancer Center and leaves with good news. Yet, I hope they leave with optimism.* Personally, I was hoping for both.

I stepped off the shuttle bus at MD Anderson and apprehensively approached the entrance. Fortunately, I did not have time for any of the bad thoughts that had plagued me the previous day. I immediately encountered a friendly smile. A man pushing a bucket with a mop sticking out waved to me as I entered.

"Good morning, Dr. Fields."

I entered the elevator and pushed the button for the eighth floor. I tried unsuccessfully to remember where I had met the man, who just greeted me.

At the check-in desk, the receptionist addressed me with a smile: "Good morning, Dr. Fields."

After just one day, all these people knew me, and I could not recall having met any of them, much less their names. I learned an important lesson that day: Pay close attention to those you encounter and greet them with a smile. You have no idea what struggles they may be facing. A friendly "hello" or "good morning" might just be the medication they need. It certainly worked for me. With each "hello," I felt a bit more relaxed and a bit of happiness and hope washed over me, even as I ventured closer and closer to what would likely not be good news.

No sooner had I sat down in the waiting room than I heard a familiar voice.

"Good morning, Dr. Fields. Please follow me."

It was the girl in the pink smock.

She led me to an examination room, where a new nurse wanted to extract more vials of blood from my already bruised arms. The blood was for a study to test the hypothesis that cytokines might be the reason for cancer-related fatigue. I recalled the form that I had signed, "Permission to Collect and Store Tissue Samples." *I assume that my clinical findings may help future patients with leukemia.*

The staff on the cancer ward knew not only my name but also that I was a professor and that I ran marathons. As the nurse prepared to collect my blood, she began sharing her experience of running the Honolulu Marathon that past December.

I never engage nurses in dialogue when they are getting ready to stick a needle into one of my veins. However, she initiated the conversation, and I braced for the inevitable. Because she was distracted due to her talking, she missed my vein. She then began twisting and turning the needle in an attempt to find blood. Being unsuccessful, she pulled the needle out a little and went back in. During all this, to my surprise (and annoyance), she did not miss a beat in talking about her first marathon. In addition, she did not seem to notice my discomfort. I briefly considered lecturing to her about the importance of focusing on her job, particularly when it involved pricking me with a needle. I kept my mouth shut and refrained from doing so. After all, she was the one holding the needle. Finally, she was successful in finding my vein and getting the blood. As she filled the last vial, I jokingly said, "I feel like I am the buffet line at a vampire convention."

My attempt at humor went right over her head. Yet, she must have thought I was serious because she began a discussion about my needing to take supplemental iron when I got home. (A deficiency of iron limits oxygen delivery to cells. This can result in fatigue, poor work performance, and decreased immunity.) At the time, I was unaware that I was only beginning to go down a long road of debilitating fatigue, impaired work performance, and reduced immunity.

Back in the waiting room, I briefly thought about this latest encounter. Yet, I could not be angry since nurses have always had a special place in my heart. Why? Mom was a nurse.

• • •

I will briefly deviate from MD Anderson and share Mom's rather extraordinary story. In the winter of 1945, Mom graduated from the University of North Carolina at Chapel Hill with an advanced degree in public health nursing. She had visited a cousin in Bushnell, Florida, and ended up staying a lifetime in Bushnell. At the age of twenty-nine, she became the first county public health nurse in Sumter County.

Mom's responsibility was to create a county health facility. A doctor drove over from Leesburg once a week to see patients. Leesburg was thirty miles away. The rest of the time, Mom was responsible for a patient's medical care.

She had many obstacles to overcome when she arrived in this Southern community. She was not only a Yankee from Ohio but also a Catholic in an area that was traditionally Baptist. Consequently, she found it difficult to gain the trust of the people she served. They viewed her as just another Northern carpetbagger.

Mom displayed a profound empathy for the destitute and eventually earned the respect of the people in the county. People referred to her as the "Angel of Mercy." Her tombstone says it best: *First Sumter County Nurse. She loved this county and its people.*

When Mom started her nursing career in Sumter County, sanitation was so bad that children were dying from hookworm infestation. At the same time, people in the area based much of their knowledge about health care on folklore. One of the traditions was to place a bracelet on the wrist or ankle of a child in order to cure worms. This obviously was not working, but Mom did not criticize or make fun of their beliefs. Instead, she agreed with the families that the bracelet might help. At the same time, she began educating them about how to build and use privies, wooden port-o-lets.

The County Sanitation Department criticized her for not insisting that they install septic tanks and indoor plumbing. She informed the sanitation department, "These people have little money and cannot afford these luxuries. You have to crawl before you can walk." Mom understood the need to work with what she had and what the people needed at the time.

Because of poor sanitation, typhoid fever and tuberculosis (TB) were widespread. Mom told us, "Back then, people with TB went to sanitariums where they remained for years. Now they can be treated at home." People working in restaurants and the local packing plant had to be tested. Mom said, "At times the line of people getting tested would extend into the yard at the clinic."

Prior to effective vaccines, polio, diphtheria, and whooping cough were prevalent. Mom watched a baby choke to death with whooping cough. She told us, "Being unable to save that baby was the worst experience I faced."

Once vaccines became available, Mom immediately attempted to initiate a vaccination program. However, people were afraid to have their children vaccinated. They viewed it as some-thing akin to witchcraft. Myths were already circulating that the vaccines were causing the illnesses.

In order to convince the community about the necessity and safety of the vaccines, Mom contacted the local newspaper and asked them to show up at the health clinic where she vaccinated Michael and me first. After that, every child in the county showed up at the health department for Mom to vaccinate them. This helped eradicate various childhood diseases such as diphtheria, whooping cough, tetanus, typhoid fever, and polio.

Back then, syringe needles were sharpened, sanitized, and reused. As a child, I remember watching Mom sharpening the needles with a sharpening stone. She then put the syringe needles in a small stainless steel tray and placed the tray in a tabletop steam sterilizer. Of course, this process left barbs on the needles. (No wonder the shots hurt so much back then! I guess that is why, to this day, I hate needles.)

People referred to Mom as the "shot lady." They still talk about how she had them pinch their noses very hard when receiving a shot. She convinced them that if they did this, they would not feel the needle. Having pinched my nose on numerous occasions, I am convinced this works.

Another health problem in Sumter County was its high infant mortality rate. People were poor and could not afford $1,000 for visits to a doctor and the hospital care. They depended on midwives to deliver their babies at home. The midwives' practice involved a lot of folklore. For example, writing an X with chalk under the pregnant woman's bed would reduce her labor pains. Another belief had to do with determining whether a baby was male or female. The pregnant woman dangled a sewing needle from a piece of thread with her right hand about an inch above her left palm. She kept both hands still and let the needle do its own thing. If the needle began to move in circles, the baby would be a girl. If the needle moved back and forth in straight lines, the baby would be a boy. The needle would not move if the woman was not pregnant.

In 1948, there were six midwives in the county. Mom began to train them in the importance of using sterile technique. She traveled to their homes and taught them how to organize a midwife pack. Importantly, she showed them how to sterilize the pack in the oven. At first, they were reluctant to do this. They questioned how they would know when the pack was in the oven long enough to be sterilized. Mom asked, "Do you eat potatoes? If so, put the pack in the oven with a potato. It will be sterilized when the potato is done." The midwives became convinced and adopted this technique.

When Mom arrived in Sumter County, most women were delivering their babies at home. There was a high death rate for premature births. Many homes in Sumter County did not have electricity. Therefore, Mom improvised and developed a home incubator that did not require electricity. She constructed a box with screens at both ends to allow air to flow. She commented with pride about that invention: "There were always whiskey bottles lying around these homes. We would fill those with hot water and stack them around the outside to help keep the premature baby warm. The family refilled the bottles as needed. Of the twenty-one babies that we incubated using this device, only one died. The baby who died was in a cold and drafty home, and it contracted pneumonia."

• • •

The cancer ward must have been on a tight schedule, since no sooner had I return to the waiting room from the latest bloodletting than I heard the girl in the pink smock say, "Dr. Phillip Fields?"

"Yes."

"Please follow me."

CHAPTER 15
The Cow Dung War

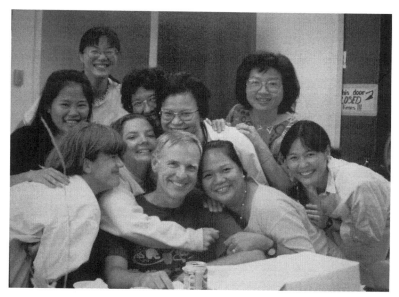

Greenwood's Lab Personnel, University of Hawaii (1994)

Never procrastinate with important things.
Time is the enemy.
Phillip Fields

The girl in the pink smock led me to a room in which a flat exam-ination table was covered with a paper sheet. There was a pillow on the table. This looked all too familiar.

Oh, (censored), I thought. *A bone marrow biopsy. Dr. Keating did not say anything about this being necessary.*

I commented that Dr. Butler had done a bone marrow biopsy in Mobile. One of Dr. Keating's associates, who was going to conduct this biopsy, said something about not getting the information they needed from the one in Mobile. A little warning would have been appreciated so that I could have mentally prepared myself for what was about to happen.

A Lidocaine injection anesthetized the skin and underlying tissues over my ilium. I can confirm that it does not work well on the bone or its connective tissue covering (the periosteum). The trocar was painless as it went through the deadened skin and fat. I swear I heard a thud when it hit my ilium. I tensed, grabbed the edges of the table, and tried to prepare myself mentally for what was to follow. First, there was pressure and then pain as Dr. Keating's associate pressed down on the trocar. Next, he rotated and pushed the trocar through the thin plate of my iliac bone and into the bone marrow cavity.

Have you ever put weight on a screwdriver and tried to penetrate an object only to have the screwdriver slip and scrape across the object? When this happened with the trocar, I recalled reading, "The tip can break off in the bone." I thought, *I should have accepted their offer of an intravenous sedation.*

Once the doctor had successfully shoved the trocar into my bone marrow cavity, he attached a syringe and extracted fluid. As he pulled back on the syringe plunger, I could feel the pressure change in the bone marrow cavity. It was not a pleasant sensation. I felt like the syringe was sucking my eyeballs down into my pelvis.

An orderly escorted me back to the waiting room in a wheelchair, where I sat and wondered what was next. I did not have to wait long to find out. The girl in the pink smock was approaching me with a chart.

"Dr. Phillip Fields?"

"Yes."

"You are free to go. They want to see you tomorrow morning at 9 o'clock."

I was again the lone passenger on the shuttle bus back to the hotel. Melancholy overwhelmed me during the bus ride. I had been alone since 2005 and had forgotten how much I loved Leslie and how much I missed seeing her each day. Yet, at the same time, I was experiencing a psychological dichotomy. There was this longing to love and to belong. However, under the circumstances, I was glad to be alone and not be a burden to anyone.

When I arrived back at the hotel, it was only 3 p.m. Since it was too early for dinner, I lay down to nap. I had lots of sleep to catch up on and a severe headache because of the bone marrow biopsy. Before I drifted off to sleep, I reflected on the nurse's conversation about the Honolulu Marathon. I have so many great memories of Hawaii—marathons, vacations, and the Greenwoods.

• • •

I first met Drs. Fred and Gill Greenwood (a husband and wife research team) in 1977 at the Annual Endocrinology meeting in San Francisco. At the time, I was doing postdoctoral studies with Dr. Lynn Larkin at the University of Florida, College of Medicine. I was presenting our research on the hormone relaxin at the meeting.

After that initial encounter, I looked forward to visiting with them at the annual meeting of the Society for the Study of Reproduction (SSR). Moreover, since Fred ran, we always managed to get in several runs together when we were attending the meetings.

My favorite memory of running with Fred occurred at the SSR meeting in Laramie, Wyoming, in 1984. It rained the entire first day, and some of the streets had turned into shallow rivers. A group of us removed our shoes and waded across one of the flooded streets. A canoe full of drunken Wyoming University Cowboys were going downhill in the rapids and almost ran us over. They each had a beer can in one hand and a cowboy hat in the other as they whooped and hollered and sang a slurred song I could not make out.

I asked our group, "Could anyone make out what they were singing?" One of the scientist in our group was from Wyoming and responded, "They were singing lyrics from the Wyoming University fight song: 'He's a high-falootin', rootin', tootin', son of a gun from ol' Wyoming!'"

How those crazy canoers managed to miss all the cars parked along the street was (and still is) a mystery to me. Obviously, their Guardian Angel was an alumnus of Wyoming University. (More like a Guardian Cowboy, perhaps.)

By the second day of the meetings, the rain had stopped and the sun had dried everything out. Fred and I, along with a group of about five more scientists, went for a run after the last scientific session. Fred led the way as we headed out of town and into cattle country. Having grown up on a ranch, the odor of fresh cow dung was a familiar and pleasant aroma to me.

The run progressed from a fun run to one of endurance. One by one, the other runners turned back. But not Fred. He kept going, and I stayed with him. Perhaps my own competitive streak came out, or maybe I was just competing with myself to see how long I could go. We had been running about ninety minutes, and it was getting dark. Finally, Fred asked, "Phil, do you think we should head back?"

I laughed a bit, as much as I could with my weariness from the run. "I thought you would never ask."

"Well, I didn't want to be the first to quit."

"Fred, I believe the first turned back sixty minutes ago."

In 1994, it was only natural that I jumped at the chance to take a research sabbatical and spend four months in the Greenwood's research lab at the University of Hawaii. Several reasons made this sabbatical special. First, I would be working with, Drs. Fred and Gill Greenwood. They not only were close friends and research collaborators but also, to me, were like family. Second, the Greenwoods were experts in sequencing the DNA of relaxin. I would learn this technique from them for my research program. Third, I would be in Hawaii (which is mostly self-explanatory). Hawaii must be similar to what Adam and Eve experienced in the Garden of Eden.

I had wanted to run the Honolulu Marathon with Fred, but I procrastinated too long and Fred died in 2000. I felt like I had lost my father.

Six years after Fred's death, I had the honor of developing and chairing a research symposium at the SSR meeting. I used that opportunity to honor Fred's contribution to the scientific community. He was one of two scientists to develop a procedure (radioimmunoassay) that allowed for the measurement of extremely low levels of hormones in the blood for the first time. This became a diagnostic tool for both researchers and clinicians when they were evaluating pathological conditions such as diabetes and infertility.

It is strange, but every time I smell fresh cow manure, I recall that run in Wyoming with my good friend. His footprints remain on my heart.

• • •

That is not my only memory invoked by the smell of fresh cow manure. When I was nine years old, I built a tree house near our barn and cattle pens. The widely spaced limbs of a large oak tree provided the perfect foundation for my construction. The bottom floor was a single room with a balcony around the outside. It looked like a fort. It was my fort.

One weekend my brother Michael, my friend Jackie, and I were playing make-believe in the tree house. Jackie was the one who showed me how to wear the football gear (Chapter 4 Related Memory). We were the U.S. Cavalry in our fort, fighting make-believe Indians. Having been victorious, we sat on the balcony floor for a lunch break. While we were enjoying our victory feast, we heard voices, got off the floor, and scanned the terrain below us. Instead of make-believe Indians, there were six very real neighborhood bullies looking up at us. They began bombarding us with dry cow dung.

Now, you would think we had the advantage in this war by having the high ground. Not so. Since cows do not climb trees, the bullies had all the ammunition. We only had what we collected off the floor of the tree house that they had thrown at us. In addition, they had more firepower. They had eleven hands versus our six. (Yes, eleven hands. You see, one bully had only one arm. He lost one by riding on the back of a tractor his father was driving while cutting underbrush. The boy fell off the tractor, and the bush hog cut one of his arms off. He was lucky that was all that the mower had removed.)

We were getting the worst of the bombardment when my brother fearlessly jumped out of the tree house. He ran around the barn with two of the larger bullies chasing after him. It was not long before the two bullies were running back with Michael chasing them. They were yelling something that I could not understand. Then I saw that my brother had both hands full of fresh cow manure. That was when I realized they were yelling, "He's throwing fresh cow (censored)." The six scattered in different directions like a flushed covey of quail.

Jackie and I climbed down from the tree house to congratulate Michael for running off the bullies. Having two hands full of fresh cow dung and no bullies left at whom he could dispatch the stuff, he threw it at Jackie and me.

I spent many evenings on weekends camping out in that tree house. The second story was the bedroom. I had covered the roof with a tarp that I could roll back and view the moon and stars through the canopy of limbs and leaves. Living in the country, the moon and stars did not have to compete with the lights from town. The sky was incredibly beautiful—a black backdrop for billions of stars that all seemed to be winking at me from millions of miles away. Then, across this canvas, God had taken a brush and made a broad yet gentle stroke that produced the Milky Way. As I studied God's masterpiece, I could hear frogs croaking in ponds that were located in the back acres. In addition, whippoorwills were chanting their namesake. Biologists named the bird onomatopoetically after its song: "Whip-poor-will, Whip-poorwill." Now, whenever I view a night sky full of stars and the moon, I am at peace. I recall my childhood and my wonderful family life, and I thank God for how blessed I have been.

CHAPTER 16

My Hardest Marathon

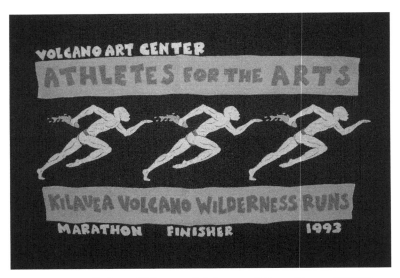

Finisher Shirt: Kilauea Volcano Marathon (1993)

"As you move outside of your comfort zone,
what was once the unknown and frightening
becomes your new normal."

Robin S Sharma[18]

I was startled from my sleep by my hotel's wakeup call. I had just taken a sixteen-hour nap. It was now Day Three at MD Anderson Cancer Center—my final day.

As I got out of bed, I felt invigorated, and I was experiencing euphoria and a renewal of hope. Why, you ask? *Today, I meet with the chief oncologist. Finally, after all the waiting, blood samples, and bone marrow biopsy, I will learn my fate.*

I was anxious to begin putting structure back into my life and to return to my comfort zone. This was something that had been missing for a year. Just maybe I would be able to start running again.

I was the only passenger on the shuttle bus that morning. The waiting room at MD Anderson was also lacking in patients. My wait was not long.

"Dr. Phillip Fields?"

"Dr. Phillip Fields?"

(It rather sounded like a whippoorwill chanting.)

"Yes."

"Please follow me."

The girl in the pink smock led me to the office of Dr. Keating. This was the last time that I would see her, and to be honest, I was somewhat glad. It was not that I begrudged her, but I was ready to say goodbye to this place.

The oncologist began, "So, how has your trip been? Have my people been treating you well?"

Before I could answer, he asked another question, "What was your hardest marathon?"

I thought, *That is a strange question.*

Nevertheless, this immediately put me at ease, since I love talking about running.

• • •

This is the long version of my answer to Dr. Keating's question. My hardest marathon was during my research sabbatical in Hawaii. During my daily runs, which started from the faculty housing, I ran past a store called the Running Room. One weekend I walked in to see what they had. There, I saw an application for a marathon on the Big Island (Hawaii) called the Kilauea Volcano Marathon. The race was limited to 150 runners.

What really caught my eye on the race form was "The World's Toughest Trail Marathon." It was a challenge I could not resist.

I immediately filled out the registration form and handed it to the store manager who was standing behind the counter. He commented, "You realize this marathon is run mostly by ultra-marathoners who use it for a training run?"

"That's okay by me. I have run many marathons." I tried to sound like I knew what I was doing, although I had an uncomfortable feeling. I wondered, *For what am I registering?*

The manager continued, "There are no aid stations for the first thirteen miles, which is across a lava field." He then showed me several types of water carriers. I purchased a belt with a pouch on the back that held a large water bottle.

As I paid for the merchandise, he told me, "There aren't any port-o-lets for the first thirteen miles either."

I jokingly responded, "I can always use my new water bottle." My comment did not elicit a response as he handed me the receipt. My final thought as I left the store was, *He is much too serious to be a runner.*

I flew to the Big Island from Oahu the day before the race. That evening I attended a pasta dinner at the mess hall of the Kilauea Military Camp. The camp was the site of the marathon start and finish. During dinner, they told us the history of the Kilauea volcano. The name means "spewing" or "much spreading." Kilauea has a long history of eruptions; the oldest uncovered lava is 2,800 years old.

The more wine we consumed, the taller the tales became by those who had run this marathon before. Before the evening's ceremony was over, I began to doubt the sanity of these repeat runners. Not to mention my own.

It was dark at 5:30 a.m. when we gathered the next morning at the military base. I scanned the runners and saw that they were wearing various types of lights (belt lanterns, head lanterns, etc.). I obviously missed that small print on the registration form and had none.

We received last-minute instructions and warnings from the race director. "Do not wander off the course. You might step through the lava crust and into a lava tube. There is no lava flow in this area, so the tubes are only hollow tunnels."

I turned to the runner next to me, "That is good news. If we fall through, we won't burn to a crisp, and they will at least be able to retrieve our bodies." Like the manager behind the counter, he was unimpressed with my humor.

The race director continued, "We have marked the course with little piles of rock, called cairns, so that you won't get lost."

This time, I turned to a runner on my other side, "That is funny. This is a lava field, and there are piles of rock everywhere."

He, too, was stoic.

I thought, *These runners are too serious. Maybe I should be more concerned about what is beginning to transpire.*

Before moving out into the lava field to toe the starting line, there was one last formality. We were required to walk through a chemical foot vat in which we scraped our shoes over wire brushes. This ritual removed any foreign plant seeds. They did not want their pristine environment contaminated with outside vegetation. Vats from previous years were an overgrown reminder of what runners can carry into the lava field.

A tropical storm had struck the island the evening before the marathon. When the race began at 6 a.m., the rain was blowing horizontally. It felt like little needles hitting my face. Yet, being a warm July, the rain and wind were rather refreshing.

After hearing all those tall tales at the pasta dinner and the warnings at the race start, I stepped onto the lave field with a bit of apprehension. Consequently, I immediately joined a group of five runners who had lights. I was hoping that between us we would spot those little piles of rock.

I noticed that they had tied themselves together by a rope and inquired, "Have you run this course before?"

"Yes, we run it every year. It is part of our ultra-marathon training."

"So what's with the rope?" I asked. I thought that, like the light, I had missed instructions about the need to bring one.

"We are a centipede."

"A centipede?"

I wondered, *Did I select the right group to follow?*

"So, what happened to your other ninety legs?" I inquired.

They greeted my sense of humor with silence. Maybe they did not get the joke: centipede, 100 legs.

The silence ensued for the next hour.

The centipede seemed to be going a tad slow for ten legs. After running for an hour, we had only completed about four and a half miles, and we were dead last. In fact, there were no other runners in sight. The sun had come up, and the rain had stopped, but the lava field had turned into a fog-covered sauna bath. The visibility was only about ten yards.

I made a quick calculation and determined it was going to take us over six hours to finish at this pace. I was used to running under four hours, and I was now going to have to make up a lot of time to do so.

After thanking the centipede for being my guide dog (uh, guide arthropod), I set out on my own. Now I was alone as I attempted to discern the cairns, which marked the course, from all the other rocks in the lava field.

The first thirteen miles were over an area of the lava field called Ka'ū Desert, an area of Hawaii Volcanoes National Park that only runners of the marathon are fortunate enough to see. It is an incredible landscape with an absence of vegetation. (The rain mixes with the sulfur dioxide and creates an acid rain with a pH 3.4, which is not very conducive for plant growth.)

With the rocky scenery, devoid of greenery, I imagined it was July 21, 1969, and I was Neal Armstrong walking on the moon. While daydreaming about space walking, I missed several cairns and ventured off the course. The race director had not explained how to detect if we were walking over a lava tube, so I was expecting to break through the crust at every step.

After considerable backtracking, careful with each step I took, I found those little piles of rock. I was again on the proper trail. Now, I slowed my pace as I attempted to spot those little piles of rock in a thick, milky, soup-like fog.

An area of Ka'ū Desert at mile 8 is called Mauna Iki, which means "little mountain." Here, several volunteers had hiked in the day before and had ridden out the tropical storm in tents to prepare and staff an aid station. This is just another example of how important volunteers are to the success of a race. This group of volunteers had truly performed a heroic deed.

They would have been even more valiant if they had carried in a port-o-let. My bladder was about to pop, but I was not about to contaminate this unspoiled terrain—or my water bottle.

The fog cleared as I exited the lava field around mile 13. The next four miles were on Hilina Pali Road and Chain of Craters Road. Here, tourists can drive and view regions of older lava flows.

Because of the fog, I had not seen any runners since leaving the centipede. Now, I began passing several. One was a woman who said, "The hard part is over. It is all downhill to the finish."

I thought, *What a strange comment. We have not been going uphill.* Then I scoffed to myself: *"World's Toughest Trail Marathon." Their description is a bit overexaggerated.*

I quickly learned that she had run this course before and was being facetious.

I turned into a picnic site, which thankfully had restrooms. Next, I took a trail into the woods. The course made a sharp right hand turn onto a jeep trail called "The Escape Route." It went straight up to the crater at a 60-degree angle. It was a six-mile ascent of a nearly 4,000-foot change in elevation. My ridicule of the course description had been premature.

The tropical storm had turned the trail into a mudslide. Runners were slipping and sliding back down the trail and taking the legs out from under any runner who ventured too close. I quickly learned not to run immediately behind anyone.

There were places where I was in the sludge up to my ankles. It was like trying to maneuver through quicksand. At various places, I used roots and vines to pull myself up the trail.

Before I reached the top of the jeep trail, mud covered me from head to toe. The color of my running shorts and singlet was no longer discernable. I could not wipe the sludge from my eyes because everything I had on was soiled. At one point, I attempted to use some large plant leaves without success.

Finally, I reached the top of Kilauea at mile 23. I stepped off the trail onto dry ground. I had so much mud on the bottom of my shoes that I felt like I was three inches taller than when the race started. I was lucky the sludge had not sucked my shoes off my feet.

The next portion of the course was a wooden walkway that took runners past Thurston Lava Tube, along the Kilauea Iki Crater rim, up and down stairs, and then over an area with sulfur gas coming up through vents in the ground.

The run finished at the Kilauea Military Camp. Of the 150 runners who had started the race (well, 145 runners and a 10-legged centipede), only 104 runners finished. My time was 4:35. I was fifty-ninth, and they presented me with a well-earned finisher's T-shirt that I have never worn. Yet, at least once a year, I remove it from its box and remember.

I never saw the centipede finish. It may have gotten its legs tangled in the rope and vines on the escape route.

• • •

I had no sooner completed the short version of the above story for Dr. Keating than he said to me, "I'm sure you must be interested in what we found. You have an aggressive form of chronic lymphocytic leukemia (CLL). How aggressive it is will depend on the results from California. As hard as what you may have thought that marathon was, it will pale in comparison to what you are about to face. You will look back at that run, and it will appear easy."

I thought, *So, this is why he asked me about my hardest marathon. He wanted to be able to relate my leukemia in a way that I will fully appreciate my condition.*

I should have asked him many questions at that exit meeting. Yet, I could think of only one: "Am I going to be able to get back to my training for the Boston Marathon?"

I believe that when confronted with bad news, we attempt to hold on to a modicum of something that makes us feel normal. Running does that for me. It opens the window to so many positive sensations. I feel the sun on my skin while my feet are hitting the pavement. There is sweating, thirst, and pain. I hear birds singing and smell automobile exhaust. If I run by a crop of ragweed, I experience an allergic reaction and my upper respiratory membranes swell. All of these are sensations of a living, breathing human being. I am running, so I must be alive. I run, therefore I am.

Dr. Keating quickly burst my bubble. "You should turn to an exercise program that is less stressful. You are going to find it fatiguing just taking out the trash, much less running a marathon. Plus, you will most likely have to start chemotherapy in three months."

Three months? Talk about a reality check. My passion had kept me company with memories and had been a respite from the reality of why I was here. Now, for the first time in these three days, this was all beginning to sink in. *I have leukemia. This is serious stuff. Dr. Keating has just moved my goalpost of normalcy back even further.*

There were the usual parting comments and exchange of pleasantries. Dr. Keating's last words were, "Contact me if you get home and think of any questions. We will contact you by e-mail after we get the results from the blood sample we sent to California. Have your oncologist in Mobile monitor your blood counts every month. The counts will determine when chemotherapy should begin."

If you ever have a friend or a family member who has to go to a cancer center, please do not let them go alone. It would have been beneficial if a friend had been with me. The friend could have taken some of the sting out of those cancer-screening tests and the discussion about housing during treatment. A friend would probably have listened more carefully and remembered what Dr. Keating said at the exit meeting. The friend also would probably have even asked questions about something other than running. Lastly, the friend would have provided a shoulder to cry on when this all began to sink in.

On the shuttle bus ride back to the hotel, I replayed the oncologist's recommendation to give up running—my passion—and I cried.

The bus driver asked me, "Is there anything I can do?"

"No. It has been a depressing three days, and I am looking forward to going home."

CHAPTER 17

Trips

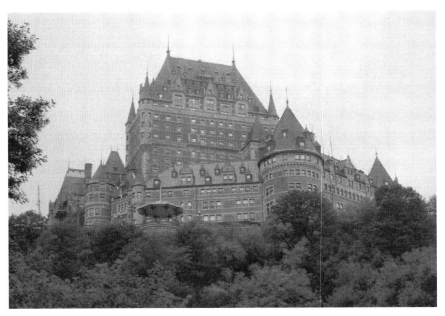

Chateau Frontenac, Quebec City (1979)

The world is a book,
and those who do not travel read only a page.

St. Augustine[19]

I spent my last evening in Houston enjoying another dinner at Ruby Tuesday. I am not sure if it was the martinis or the mental exhaustion from the previous three days, but I slept well that night.

The next morning, I packed my truck and got on the road for Mobile. An eight-hour drive lay ahead of me—too much time to think endlessly about the past three days. I did not want to preoccupy myself with thoughts about how leukemia would change my life. There would be plenty of time for that when I got home from this trip. Besides, there were still too many uncertainties. I had made a huge mistake by not making a list of questions to discuss with Dr. Keating.

I can sum the trip up as three days of tests, endless memories, and less than thirty minutes visiting with the chief oncologist and my only concern was about being able to run. Consequently, I did not know much more about my condition than I did before that trip.

• • •

Trips have always been a part of my life. I was five years old when I went on my first adventure. My parents loaded up our 1950 Oldsmobile touring sedan with my brother, our suitcases, and myself. We were on our way to Defiance, Ohio, to visit Mom's parents and her four sisters. She actually had five sisters—Amy, Mary, Sophia, Sylvia, and Kathryn. I never had a chance to meet the youngest, Kathryn. She died in 1933 at the age of twenty-four from Hodgkin's lymphoma.

Mom recognized the importance of travel in shaping our minds and bringing our family together. Before we got on the road, Mom told Michael and me, "Throughout your lives, you will be taking trips. What you get out of the trips will be left up to you."

With our naive interpretation, we began collecting mementos from each family trip. We labeled our treasures to remind us where they came from and displayed them on a shelf in our bedrooms. Michael collected model Civil War cannons from all the various Civil War battlefields we visited. I collected rocks.

Michael and I spent many of our summer vacations in Atlanta, Georgia, visiting our two cousins and our uncle, Dr. James H. Steele. Jim, as we called him, was a great mentor and reinforced what Mom had been telling us regarding the importance of a college education.

Jim's résumé alone was enough to inspire us to reach for more. Dr. Steele was a Doctor of Veterinary Medicine with a degree from Michigan State and a master's degree in public health from Harvard University. In 1947, he established and was the first director of the Veterinary Division of the Center for Disease Control and Prevention (CDC) in Atlanta. He was the first Assistant Surgeon General for Veterinary Affairs and the Deputy Assistant Secretary for Health and Human Services at the rank of Admiral, two stars.

Dr. Steele is the architect of and was, until his death, an advocate for *One World, One Health, and One Medicine*. This health care system incorporates various medical specialties. Veterinarians, doctors, and people in various public health specialties work together to address health care issues around the world.

Among Dr. Steele's many awards were the XIIth International Veterinary Congress Prize from the American Veterinary Medical Association (AVMA), the Surgeon General's Medallion, and the Medal of Merit from the World Organization for Animal Health. He was an impressive man, a true pioneer. For more about the incredible journey of Dr. Steele, read the biography of him, *One Man, One Medicine, One Health: The James H. Steele Story*, by Dr. Craig Carter.

During those summers, we saw the unimaginable wonders that were available through education. World dignitaries were always dining at our uncle's house. Jim's wife Aina was a wonderful aunt and a great cook. During these meals, we sat quietly and listened to discussions about various world health problems. The visiting dignitaries talked about attempts to eradicate diseases that were prevalent in their countries, for example, hoof and mouth disease, malaria, typhoid fever, and rabies.

After dinner, either Jim or his houseguests treated us to a slideshow of their travels. Michael and I sat and watched in awe. There were slides of the Nile River, pyramids, camels, and crocodiles. We saw the Great Wall of China, the Eiffel Tower, Mount Kilimanjaro, lions, and elephants. There were slides of the Kremlin Palace, the Taj Mahal, the Amazon River, and anacondas.

For two young boys from Sumter County, Florida, these slide shows opened windows to so many places in a world that we had not imagined existed. We were transfixed.

• • •

When Michael and I were older (high school and then college), we vacationed in North Carolina with Mom. She had a cabin in Franklin, North Carolina. There, Michael and I joined a mountain climbing and kayaking club. One summer I met some real North Carolina hillbillies–and I use the word *hillbillies* with affection. They invited me to join them one evening in a backwoods cabin for some friendly poker. They picked me up at Mom's cabin and blindfolded me during the ride to their cabin. I had seen this done before in gangster movies, and the outcome was not favorable.

I inquired, "Is this blindfold really necessary?" They obviously sensed the nervousness in my voice and began teasing me. At least I think they were.

"If we thought you could lead the Feds to our hideout, we would have to shoot you and bury you in these woods. No one would ever find you."

We did not travel far on the paved road when we turned onto a path that I can only describe as washboard-like. After what seemed like an hour, the car came to a halt. My heart began to race.

When they removed my blindfold, I understood the comment about no one finding me. I was in the backwoods of nowhere. Their log cabin resembled something I had seen as a youngster watching the TV show, *Daniel Boone*, on Saturday mornings. The lodging came complete with hound dogs and a shed with a huge moonshine still. The reason for the blindfold was now evident.

One by one, other vehicles began arriving, and the host introduced me to those who would be joining us for the card game. As one of the men shuffled the deck of cards, our host brought out a jug of their home brew and set it on the table with a thud: moonshine. That was the best tasting alcohol I have experienced. It was as clear as spring water, as smooth as silk, and it had the kick of a mule that snuck up on me.

We drank until the jug was empty. My wallet was also empty by the time they took me back to Mom's cabin. Moonshine and cards are not compatible companions, at least for me.

• • •

In 1982, after Michael and I had begun working full time, we took Mom on a tour of Italy (Venice, Florence, Pisa, Rome, and Pompeii). In Florence, Michael and I presented our research at an international research conference. Mom was exceptionally proud of us as she sat in the audience and listened to our talks. At one point in the meeting, she became upset when she felt another scientist was questioning my results in a less than professional manner. I could hear her comments from the podium where I stood and presented.

Afterwards, I introduced Mom to some of the various scientists—not those with whom she was perturbed. One commented, "So this is the lady in the audience who was standing up for you."

We took Mom with us to SSR meetings in Canada (Vancouver, Quebec City, and Ontario). After the meeting in Ontario, we visited Niagara Falls.

• • •

Leslie and I took Mom on a trip to Europe in 1988. Our first stop was England. A funny thing happened on our way from the airport to our bed and breakfast. We took the scenic and romantic form of travel to our hotel: the double-decker red bus. While the bus was moving, the ticket agent sat in an area in the back of the bus on the lower deck. When the bus stopped, he got off to sell tickets. While I purchased tickets, Leslie and Mom quickly boarded the bus and, unknown to me, tossed their luggage in the ticket agent's area before hurrying upstairs to find seats. As I started up the stairs with my suitcase, a booming voice called out behind me, "What the bloody hell? Whose luggage is this? This ain't no bloody truck."

I struggled up the stairs with five pieces of luggage. At the top, Mom and Leslie were in the last two available seats, laughing along with the other tourists.

In London, we visited the National Gallery, London Bridge, and the Tower of London. We lucked out and got the last three tickets (seated together) for *The Phantom of the Opera*.

We took the ferry across the English Channel and traveled to Paris. There, we sat on the lawn beneath the Eiffel Tower, ate lunch (fresh bread, cheese, and wine), and watched people.

I had purchased our lunch items at an "off the beaten path" market where the owner only spoke French. The eyes of the woman behind the counter dilated as I attempted to pay while reading from a translation book. She graciously waited on me in spite of my annihilation of her beautiful language with my broken Southern accent.

From Paris, we traveled to Brussels and then to Bruges, an enchanting Flemish city with cobblestone streets lined with hanging flower baskets. The Dijver canal snakes through town. They refer to this beautiful medieval city as the "Venice of the North."

In Belgium, we boarded a train for Amsterdam. There, I managed to get us lost on a self-guided walking tour while we were looking for windmills. After leading us about aimlessly for some time, I looked at the city map at Leslie's insistence. After doing so, I plotted a shortcut back to our bed and breakfast residence and again got us lost. Night descended on us while we were in the center of the famous red-light district. While we walked along the streets, we watched as people sold and bought drugs and other items in the open. At one point, we turned around to find that Mom was several blocks behind us. She was staring at a scantily dressed mannequin in a window of a shop that had a red light over the front door. We hurried back to get her.

"These mannequins are so lifelike," she commented.

"They are alive, Mom. It is time to go."

We came across a police officer on a horse, who led us safely away from the area. Of course, Mom would have preferred to linger longer in order to watch the people.

From Amsterdam, we traveled north by train to Alkmaar, the City of Cheese (**Chapter Related Memory: Choo Choo Train.** The story is at the end of the chapter).

Not many daughters-in-law would agree to share their vacation travels with their mothers-in-law. I have always been grateful that Leslie allowed Mom to experience those magnificent sights. Now, instead of reflecting on Mom's final days in the hospital that would happen later, I remember the great travels we shared through the years.

Every trip was full of wonderful memories. We visited famous buildings, historical sites, national parks, art galleries, and prehistoric collections. In addition, we enjoyed going to operas and musicals, eating unusual foods, and best of all, spending family time together.

Many decades ago, I sat in the den at my uncle's home in Atlanta, watching a slideshow. My desire for travel was stimulated, and I have yet to quench that thirst.

However, it was January 2008 and I was returning from the MD Anderson Cancer Center in Houston, Texas. This was a trip I would just as soon not have taken. Yet, my journey with leukemia was just beginning.

Chapter Related Memory: Choo, Choo Train

From Amsterdam, we traveled north by train to Alkmaar, the City of Cheese.

I have enjoyed trains since I was a young boy listening to Dad's stories. When Dad was twenty-one, he ran an engine in the ammunition yard in Baltimore during World War I. Later, he ran a locomotive in the lime-rock mines in Florida.

Mom's parents emigrated from Czechoslovakia, went through Ellis Island, and ended up in Defiance, Ohio. Her father had a cornfield next to the train rails. A coal-powered engine pulled cars past several times each day. Michael and I would run into the cornfield to watch the train go by. It was one of those large black engines with wheel sets and connecting rods. A large bell was on top of the engine.

The thick, black, billowing smoke with its pungent coal smell and the ringing of the bell has always been a special memory.

CHAPTER 18
Mastering Kiai

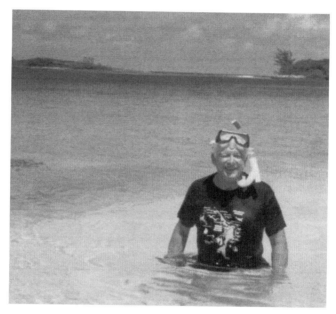

Snorkeling with Grant, Pensacola (1994)

You have power over your mind, not outside events.
Realize this, and you will find strength.

Marcus Aurelius[20]

During the drive back to Mobile, Alabama, I recalled the oncologist's recommendation not to run. I have known runners who had to give up running for various reasons and wondered how they dealt with it.

Now, the same question confronted me: *How do I give up my passion and continue to live happily? Not being able to run will make my diagnosis more than life changing. It will make it life shattering.*

• • •

Injuries have forced me to stop running a couple of times, but only temporarily.

While doing a postdoctorate at the University of Florida (1976–1980), I trained in karate. The style was Cuong Nhu. At that time, karate was my passion.

From five years of training, I developed many of the traits that prepared me for running a marathon: confidence, discipline for training, and mental focus.

My sensei (teacher or mentor) was Ngo Dong. In addition to self-defense, he taught me how to dig deep into my kiai, my inner strength. He had a way of getting me to accomplish things that I perceived were beyond my limits. Accessing one's kiai is something that is necessary to complete a marathon. It is also something that I would definitely have to exploit after my trip to MD Anderson.

When I moved to Mobile, Alabama (1980), I immediately looked for a karate dojo to train. No one taught Cuong Nhu, so I studied Taekwondo. On a Saturday in 1983, I was taking the Taekwondo black belt test. Following a jump-spinning foot strike to break boards, I planted my foot incorrectly when I landed. There was a loud pop, followed by a sharp pain in my right knee, which instantly swelled to the size of two softballs. I had torn my right anterior cruciate ligament and right medial meniscus.

Back then, orthopedic surgeons recommended that letting the knee self-heal would be the best option. (The gold standard for cruciate ligament and meniscus repairs would not occur until the 1990s.)

Karate was no longer in my future and, needing something to fill the void, I took up swimming. It became immediately apparent that I was not very good at swimming laps. My wake was like that of a fully loaded barge that a tugboat was pushing down the Mississippi River. People who swam in a lane next to me one day would move over several lanes the next day. A shark would definitely zero in on me as a floundering injured prey (**Chapter Related Memory: Swimming with Sharks.** The story is at the end of the chapter).

Yet, after one month, I was swimming a mile every day in twenty-five minutes. I can honestly say that they were the most boring twenty-five minutes. The pool never changed; the crack I saw on the bottom was there every day. There were no seasonal changes; the water temperature at the YMCA was always 87 degrees Fahrenheit.

After a year, swimming laps was not something I wanted to continue doing, so I took up running again. One year later, in 1984, I ran my first marathon (Pleasure Island Marathon) and immediately developed a new passion.

For twenty years after my knee injury healed itself, I ran without experiencing any knee pain. Then, in December 2004, without any warning, my knee became too painful to run on. The old karate injury had reemerged. In April 2005, I had surgery to repair my right anterior cruciate ligament, as well as the medial and lateral menisci. The orthopedic surgeon, Dr. Al Pearsall, also shaved the undersurface of my patella in order to remove the rough areas.

This new hiatus from running revealed that my passion and my physical and mental well-being were connected. I had apparently become a running addict, and withdrawal was a very unpleasant experience. I was moody, became angry easily, did not sleep well, and was constantly snacking. You might say I was depressed. Fortunately, the recovery period was only six months, and I began running again, or I did something that resembled running.

The YMCA had a 1/8-mile outdoor track. At first, one extremely uncomfortable lap around the track was all my knee could tolerate. I began to have serious doubts about being able to run again. I thought, *Maybe I just need to work harder and dig deeper into my kiai.* As the sensei told us each day at karate, "You need discipline."

Slowly and painfully, I added a lap each week until I was running one mile without stopping. I then switched to the half-mile outdoor clay track at the YMCA and worked up to three miles. The discomfort eventually disappeared, and my confidence returned.

My return to running after surgery had required more inner strength than I imagined was in me. My sensei had said, "You will never fully master your kiai. There will always be greater heights to scale, greater challenges to overcome, and greater focus required." His words definitely applied to my postsurgery running.

By December 2006, two years after my knee surgery, my long runs were eighteen miles and I had completed my speed work program. This was the same program I had used for my two other qualifiers for the Boston Marathon. I was fifty-nine years old and needed to run a marathon at a nine-minute pace in order to qualify for Boston.

My plan was to qualify at the February 2007 Mardi Gras Marathon. In spite of the time off for knee surgery, I was still on the schedule that I had created after the 2004 Boston Marathon. First, I would do a training run, the First Light Marathon in Mobile.

At this point in my story, I have come full circle, back to where my story began in Chapter 1 with the First Light Marathon and my trip to MD Anderson Cancer Center. My journey with leukemia was just beginning. Attempts to master my kiai would prove even more difficult with my new companion, leukemia.

Chapter Related Memory: Swimming with Sharks

People who swam in a lane next to me one day would move over several lanes the next day. A shark would definitely zero in on me as a floundering injured prey.

In 1978, doctors diagnosed my brother Michael with a tumor in his cerebellum. He went to North Florida Regional Hospital for brain surgery. Fortunately, the tumor was benign. It was also fortuitous that Doti Holmes was his nurse. We began dating, and she became my third love.

Doti's parents lived in Pensacola. It would require a book to convey how special her mother and father were.

Her father, Dr. Grant Holmes, was a dermatologist and an avid snorkeler. After I moved to Mobile in 1980, I joined him one weekend and was immediately hooked on the sport. Every Tuesday during the summer, I drove to Pensacola and spent the night at the Holmes' home. Grant and I would sit up late into the evening drinking Scotch and talking about life. My Scotch was on the rocks; Grant poured milk over his.

We would get up early the next morning and drive to Pensacola Beach as the sun was coming up. At the water's edge,

Grant would scan the ocean for a flock of seagulls hovering over the water. The birds indicated that a school of fish was below the surface. That would be our destination.

Of course, when we entered the water, we did not know if we would see anything. Sometimes the algae were so thick that we could not see twelve inches in front of us. There was nothing scarier than a four-foot crevalle jack appearing out of nowhere and swimming past my face. At least it was not a shark. (Yet.)

In July and August, when the water was warm, jellyfish were so numerous that our bodies would become numb from the stings. Yet, regardless of the condition of the water, Grant would enter the ocean and swim out toward the horizon. His passion was being in the salt water, mask facing down, snorkel up, and flippers ever so slowly propelling him along.

On one particular fall morning in 1981, the crisp air was especially refreshing, and the water was clear. There was not a cloud in the sky, but there was a distant flock of seagulls. We both knew without speaking that those squawking birds were our destination. The seagulls were also a beacon for some fish with some rather large fins that were cutting through the ocean surface like a knife through butter.

Grant was excited as we entered the water, but seeing those large fins in the water, I was apprehensive. I asked Grant, "Do you think we should be doing this?" Grant's response was, "In all my years snorkeling, I have never seen a shark. This will be an once-in-a-lifetime experience for us."

I was concerned that sharks might cut short our lifetime or, at the very least, our appendages. Nevertheless, there was no way I was letting Grant go snorkeling alone.

We saw a magnificent school of fish. There were baitfish and some rather large king mackerel. There were also the owners of those huge fins—bull sharks. Bull sharks like to feed in the shallow waters. Consequently, they are one of the most frequent attackers of swimmers.

Grant guided us right into the middle of the baitfish and sharks. At first, the sharks were more interested in the tasty mackerel than in us. It was a spectacular feeding frenzy as these sharks sliced through the fish like a food processor.

Soon the sharks began to find us more attractive than the mackerel. They began gliding past us within touching distance. Desiring to keep all my limbs, I did not attempt to stroke the sharks. I can still recall their large white eyes and gaping mouths with beautiful rows of serrated teeth. I desperately needed to pee. Not wanting to attract any more attention to myself, I refrained from doing so.

When Grant motioned that we should slowly get out of there, I did not need a second prompting. Now, my tugboat-like wake was unwise. I attempted to exit with the least amount of motion.

Some years later (1997), I attended Grant's funeral service. I felt as if someone were ripping out a part of my heart as the family released his ashes in the same spot where we had gone snorkeling with the sharks. I have not worn my mask, snorkel, and flippers since, although I suspect that Grant is still snorkeling in Heaven's ocean. The water is probably as clear as it was on that day with the sharks. He no doubt has a piece of algae behind each ear, a reminder of his snorkeling days at Pensacola Beach.

What became of Doti, my third love? When I moved to Mobile in 1980, Doti gave up nursing and moved to Mobile. She began working toward a degree in chemical engineering. Our relationship was simply poor timing. I was a new faculty member in the College of Medicine at the University of South Alabama. My focus was on promotion and tenure, without which I felt too insecure in my ability to support Doti. This was foolish on my part since she was quite capable of supporting herself. In the end, she grew tired of waiting in a relationship that did not appear to be going anywhere.

I miss Doti, too.

SECTION II:

RUNNING MARATHONS WITH LEUKEMIA

CHAPTER 19

Wait and Watch

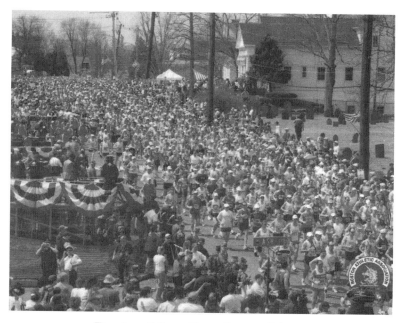

Boston Marathon Start (2004)

*I have learned now that while those who speak
about one's miseries usually hurt,
those who keep silent hurt more.*

C. S. Lewis[21]

Up to this point, I have described how I developed a passion for running marathons. Now, I will share my battle with leukemia as it attempted to deprive me of this passion and impede my efforts to return to the most prestigious marathon of them all, the Boston Marathon. This is the beginning of my long road back to Boston.

When I returned home from Houston, thoughts would not stop rolling around my head, such as, *There is no more denial; I have leukemia. This is not a ghost in a bad dream that will go away when I wake up. This is not a teacher, standing behind me, who will go away if I do not look* (**Chapter Related Memory: The Chalk Holder**. The story is at the end of the chapter).

I returned to work on Monday and immersed myself in the biomedical library to learn more about leukemia. I read everything from the history of leukemia to the cell markers that my B-lymphocytes expressed.

The word *leukemia* comes from two Greek words, *Leucos* and *Heima*, which translates to "white blood." Leukemia is a blood cancer that presents as an uncontrolled increase in abnormal white blood cells. These abnormal white cells were crowding out and compromising the function of the normal white cells, which is to fight bacterial infections, and that of normal red cells, which is to transport oxygen.

Usually, leukemia goes undetected until the patient visits the doctor with symptoms. Symptoms can range from fatigue, frequent infections, bone pain, chills, fever, sweating, bruising easily, swollen lymph nodes, an enlarged liver or spleen, and weight loss. Fatigue and enlarged lymph nodes were my only symptoms initially. Had I not been training for the Boston Marathon, there is no telling how long my leukemia would have gone undetected.

I read about those strange cell markers on my lymphocytes that indicated I had an aggressive form of chronic lymphocytic leukemia (CLL).

Here is the *Reader's Digest* version of how this works scientifically. Every cell in the body has various normal cell surface markers, called "proteins." One of the proteins is CD38, which is normally low on mature B-lymphocytes but was elevated on mine. CD38 supports proliferation and survival of B-cells on their way to becoming neoplastic. In other words, this protein promotes tumor growth.

A second marker is ZAP-70. T-cells, which fight viral infections, normally express this marker, and it promotes the positive action of these cells. Its aberrant expression on B-cells, in a certain population of patients with CLL, promotes uncontrolled cell growth and enhances cell migration. Thus, these abnormal cells are metastatic. CLL patients who are positive for ZAP-70 have an average survival rate of five to seven years, whereas CLL patients who are negative for ZAP-70 have an average survival rate of more than twenty-five years.

Third, my B-cells had the un-mutated form of the gene IgV_h, an immunoglobulin that is the business end of the lymphocyte. This sounds backward, but the un-mutated form is bad. Normally, this immunoglobulin undergoes a mutation to make the lymphocyte an active immune cell. Being un-mutated, mine are nonfunctional, worthless, and clogging up my vascular system. They identified this marker in the sample that the oncologist had sent to California.

Lastly, my serum β_2 microglobulin was elevated. This is a marker for tumor burden.

The literature confirmed the final report that I had received from MD Anderson. A combination of elevated CD38 and ZAP-70, and the un-mutated form of IgV_h are predictors of a poor prognosis, or poor "outcome." The word *outcome* was said much too often by doctors, nurses, and patients at the MD Anderson

Cancer Center. By the third day, I felt like Pavlov's dog—someone would say *outcome*, and I would sense an electrical impulse coursing through my body. To this day, the word outcome gives me chills, as if a ghost is passing through my aura. Something about the word causes me to pause and think about my mortality.

I needed a bucket with which to drink from this well of knowledge that I had uncapped in the library, not a small ladle. Delving into the realm of blood oncology was creating more questions than answers: *Why is there only a five- to seven-year life expectancy? Why do leukemia patients die? What symptoms will I experience when time is running out?*

One statistic really caught my eye. According to the National Cancer Institute, doctors diagnose 45,000 new cases of CLL each year, and 22,000 CLL patients die each year.

Dr. Keating had said, "Chemotherapy will begin when your white cell count reaches a certain level and, importantly, when their number begins doubling." (I will explain why in Chapter 25 when I discuss chemotherapy.) Thus, every month I went to the Mitchell Cancer Institute in Mobile for more blood to be drawn and for the oncologist to monitor my blood cell counts. My red blood cell count decreased below normal. Fortunately, my white blood cell count only increased slowly and was nowhere close to doubling between blood samplings.

The three months came and went without me requiring chemotherapy. The monthly blood sampling persisted, and the wait and watch continued. While waiting for the inevitable chemotherapy, I did not want to change my routine more than was necessary. Doing so would be a reminder that things were not normal. More than that, I did not want people pitying me. Even though I was hurting on the inside, I tried not to let my feelings show on the outside. My attempts to do so became increasingly difficult.

This new companion, cancer, which was growing inside me, was creating massive mood swings. Unfortunately, I had nothing to create a diversion for myself from the cancer, thoughts of chemotherapy, or those of death. The oncologist had taken away my passion.

It was hard to tell if my behavior was affecting those around me. I hoped it was not. I have never been to a psychiatrist or been diagnosed with depression, so I can only assume that is what I experienced. Moreover, it was debilitating. All I wanted to do was sleep, but even then, sleep did not come easily with a five- to seven-year life expectancy flashing like a bright red neon sign in my apartment at night.

There were times during that initial depression when I needed to talk to someone. I turned to a colleague at work who was a close friend, Dr. Susan LeDoux. She was among a handful of people I had initially informed about my condition on a need-to-know basis. Importantly, she was a good listener and someone to whom I could convey my deepest feelings. I am not sure that I could have climbed out of that initial abyss without her help.

• • •

I began waking up in the middle of the night with my bed soaked in sweat. The oncologist said that one of the symptoms of leukemia would be night sweats, caused by a rise in body temperature. I believe mine were because of the nightmares that I was experiencing. I kept dreaming about those leukemia patients I had seen in the waiting room at MD Anderson Cancer Center. The waiting room was full of hairless, emaciated patients wearing facemasks. Most were undergoing chemotherapy, and they looked as if they had just gotten off a bus from Auschwitz. I overheard stories about their latest infection that put them in the hospital because they were immunocompromised.

I began thinking, *Is this what I have in my future? If chemotherapy is going to ravage my body like that, I had better be in good physical shape going into it.*

Yet, the oncologist had told me, "Exercise, but don't push yourself too hard. Stop when your body tells you to stop. Stick to things like walking or swimming or riding a bike. Do not run."

Running is the one thing that keeps me sane. It is my psychiatric couch. Leslie had once told me, "Please don't miss a day of running. When you do, you are too grumpy to be around." Yet, I followed the oncologist's advice for almost three months.

I do not remember where, but I once read, "It is what we do when confronted with bad news that establishes who we are and what we will be from that point on." I made a decision: *To hell with a five-to-seven year prognosis. To hell with "outcome." If leukemia is going to kill me, let me at least die doing what I love: running. It is who I am.*

After a week of running, there was no unusual bruising, bleeding, or ruptured spleen. The only downside was the debilitating fatigue. To this day, the fatigue leaves me not only physically but also mentally and emotionally exhausted. Additional sleep does not relieve these symptoms. When the alarm goes off in the morning, I feel like I have already run ten miles. I get up, shave, and brush my teeth. I then lay down and rest. Most mornings I do not even want to get out of bed, but I do.

By the time I arrive at work, my energy meter is on zero. It is hard to concentrate, and everyday activities that I once took for granted are a major physical strain. Of course, the fatigue only gets worse as the day progresses.

A lot of discipline is required to get out of bed each morning. Even more discipline is required to run in the afternoon after working all day.

. . .

Why is fatigue associated with leukemia? My low red blood cell count and low hemoglobin are most likely the major factors. After all, red blood cells transport oxygen to all the cells in our body. Without sufficient oxygen, our organs and muscles do not properly function. Anemic patients feel fatigue and shortness of breath. Shortness of breath would become a major problem for me later.

Whatever the cause for the fatigue, they have given it a fancy name: cancer-related fatigue (CRF). The medical profession abbreviates everything. I guess doctors want to keep their patients in the dark. A patient will not mind paying $150 for a diagnosis of CRF. However, charge them $150 for a diagnosis of fatigue, and they likely will not return. They did not need a doctor to tell them that they were tired.

. . .

In spite of the fatigue, I was excited to be running again. I felt normal, and the embers of my passion were aglow. I started sleeping better, and I was feeling confident that I could beat leukemia. Importantly, running took my mind off the time bomb that was ticking inside me. The dark cloud of depression cleared, and the sun was shining bright again. I just needed a goal to keep the sky clear. Consequently, I did something crazy. At least, my oncologist said it was. I registered for the February 2009 Pensacola Marathon. I now had a goal that made leukemia inconsequential, at least in my mind.

...

(My library work led me to some resources that I recommend to anyone who wants to read about their particular type of cancer. One website in particular provides information for every type of cancer: cancer.gov. On another website, practiceupdate.com, you can sign up to receive a free newsletter via e-mail. Articles discuss the latest medical discoveries for all forms of cancer. I signed up for articles about chronic lymphocytic leukemia.)

Chapter Related Memory: The Chalk Holder

This is not a teacher, standing behind me, who will go away if I do not look.

It was 1954, and I was in the third grade. I was standing in line at the water fountain on my way to recess when a fourth-grader cut in front of me. I shoved him out of the way and gave him a sign with my middle finger.

God has not blessed me with proper timing. My third-grade teacher was standing behind me and was a witness to the entire incident. The next thing I knew, she was dragging me by my ear to the classroom. *Looks like I will not be going to recess today,* I speculated.

The classroom had chalkboards on three of the walls. Large windows filled the fourth wall. My punishment at subsequent recess periods was to write on the chalkboards, "I will not make signs with my fingers." I could not go to recess until I had written this 500 times.

Each time I filled the chalkboards with my writing, the teacher counted the lines. She kept a tally at the top right corner of one of the boards. At one point, I considered changing the number but wisely did not do so.

The funny thing is, at the time, I had no idea what giving the finger meant. It would be months before Jackie Huggins would explain it to me. Of course, he is the one who showed me how to make the sign to begin with. (This is the same Jackie Huggins in the football gear story; Chapter 4 Related Memory)

A chalk holder hung from a hook beside each chalkboard. The teacher used this device to create straight lines on the chalkboard for us to write on. It had a wooden handle and five wire chalk holders. While the teacher patrolled the playground, I loaded up the holder with chalk. While transcribing five lines at a time, I thought, *I will finish these 500 lines before the week is out.*

It is strange how I can sense when someone is glaring at me from behind. I remember thinking to myself, *Maybe she will go away if I do not look.*

However, she did not go away. I was required to erase the number in the corner indicating the lines completed and start over. I do not remember going to recess during the rest of the third grade.

CHAPTER 20
Mind Over Body

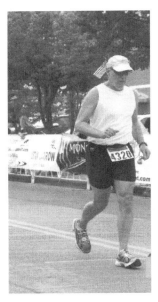

Pensacola Marathon (2009)

Wait. Why am I thinking about Krispy Kremes?
We're supposed to be exercising.

Meg Cabot[22]

Two friends, Will Wright and Don Withers, said they were going
to drive over early Sunday morning and run the Pensacola
Marathon. I had booked a hotel room within walking distance

of the start/finish line, so I offered to let them share my room on Saturday night.

On Saturday afternoon, we went to the packet pickup to get our race bibs and marathon T-shirts. Don talked nonstop; Don and Will had run over 100 marathons together, and Don had a story about each one. I learned that they were both members of something called the "50 States Marathon Club." Both of them had run a marathon in every state. For years, they had been running a marathon each month and using that as their long training runs.

(Looking back, I now see that this conversation planted the seeds for my next goal. I will explain shortly.)

After getting our race packets, we went to an Italian restaurant in the mall for a premarathon spaghetti dinner and a sharing of more stories. I heard about their running the triple at Lake Tahoe, which consisted of running a marathon on each of three consecutive days. Another race was the Disney challenge: running a half marathon on Saturday and a full marathon on Sunday.

Back at the hotel, the stories continued until we finally turned the lights out and went to sleep.

It was 5 a.m. on Sunday, and my clock alarm went off. The start of the Pensacola Marathon was just two hours away. The training was behind me, and there was nothing more to do. Now all that remained was a final mental preparation and breakfast.

My favorite premarathon meal is two Krispy Kreme donuts. They get me through the first five miles of the race without hunger pains. Power Gel packs get me through the rest of the race. I am not convinced the gel packs provide much energy, but they do take the edge off my hunger pains.

While standing at the starting line, I contemplated what was about to transpire. I wondered, *What will it be like running 26.2 miles with leukemia? How much more will this marathon extract from me than any of the previous twenty-six marathons I ran when I was healthy?* In most of my eighteen-mile training runs with leukemia, I would hit the wall by mile 6. Then it would take all of my mental fortitude to complete the last twelve miles. My final thought was, *Will I be able to finish?*

I was startled from my musings by the sound of the gun. The marathon had begun. I was fearful of what lay ahead.

The Pensacola Marathon was two loops. The second loop was a repeat of the first loop. The first two miles were relatively flat. I began running at a ten-minute pace, the pace at which I had trained. The next three miles were up a steady incline. The incline was not steep, but it was continuous enough to deplete my scant energy reserves. I reached the crest of the incline feeling exhausted and realized that I still had twenty-one more miles to go—a disheartening revelation.

The voice of uncertainty was rearing its ugly head. I started focusing on anything that would take my mind off the pain and the nagging feeling of self-doubt. This was not the time for negative thoughts. Instead, I focused on my form. *Are my breathing and cadence coordinated and steady? Are my arms relaxed and swinging straight, forward and backward by my sides?* I kept reminding myself, *Conserve energy, conserve energy.* I scanned the course for anything that would give me happy thoughts. Up ahead was a Pizza Hut, and I thought about my favorite type of pizza: *a thin crust, with pepperoni. Hmm...Maybe I will get one for dinner tonight.*

The next five miles were up steep hills. There was lots of running up, up, up. As I reached the top of the last hill in that stretch, I found myself laughing at the fatigue I was experiencing. In some sick way, the moment was incredibly comical. I was breathing but did not seem to be taking in any oxygen. My legs felt like someone had strapped an anvil to each of them. My brain commanded them to move, but they were not responding. I had never before felt anything so bizarre. Yet, making it to the top of that last hill generated the most amazing feeling of accomplishment. I had just experienced more discomfort thrown at my body than ever before, and I was still moving forward. My excitement was short-lived when I realized that I was less than half way to the finish line. The thought of running those hills again was not pleasant. My mind and body battled as I approached the point for a decision, the half marathon finish.

Keep going, my mind shouted.

Quit! Screamed my body, the fatigue overtaking it.

If you quit, you will not be able to force yourself to finish a marathon again, was my mind's final response.

That last thought inspired me to continue. I told myself, *If I quit, stopping halfway through this marathon, it will be an end of my dream to run the Boston Marathon again. I have trained very hard for this. If I cannot force myself to complete this one, I will not likely attempt another.*

For better or worse, I passed the half marathon finish line and continued running. My mind was shouting, *Run, Fields, run.*

During my second time running up the steady three-mile incline, a runner came up beside me and said, "I hope you do not mind my running right behind you. You seem like you know what you are doing and have been keeping a steady pace. I am going to try and follow you to the finish line." I laughed to myself as I thought, *This runner thinks I have been keeping a steady pace and wants me to pace him to the finish. I wonder if he can keep up with an ambulance because that is what I may need to finish this marathon.* I responded, "No problem. Maybe we can help each other to the finish line."

Now I could not stop, and I had to maintain this pace since someone was counting on me. This was a motivating force. It kept me focused on something other than the hills that were lurking.

By mile 18, I was beginning to run up the hills a second time. They seemed steeper than the first time. My calves burned, and I could not breathe. I wanted to stop and walk up those hills so much, but I kept telling myself, *I am too close to the finish line to give up now.*

As much as I thought I had suffered in the first half, I was revising my definition of "agony" as I ran up those hills a second time. Little did I know that in the not-too-distant future, I would look back at this marathon and say, *Pensacola was so easy.*

I prayed as I ran, *Just let me cross the finish line. I do not want people talking after my death.* I could almost hear someone saying, *Poor guy, he was so close to completing that marathon.* Then someone else adding, *But at least he tried.* I hate pity, especially when I am the recipient.

By mile 23, the only thing that kept me moving was my passion. *I could not. No, I would not let leukemia take it from me.*

Once I reached Palafox Street, the course was a gradual descent into the downtown area. I felt like surging but remembered I was more than two miles from the finish line. I was too close to do something stupid and collapse before the end of the race. I kept telling myself, *Keep steady, keep steady.*

Next, there was a left-hand turn and a run through Seville Square and Historic Downtown Pensacola. The finish was still a lot of twists and turns away. I was glad I had not surged on Palafox Street; it appeared that the finish line had become a moving target. The closer I got to it, the more it seemed to move away. The course was no longer definable, and the finish line appeared to be a mirage.

I was jolted from my exhausted mantra (*Keep steady*) by the cheering at the finish line. I knew that the cheering was not for me, but I imagined it was. One last turn and I saw the finish line at the end of a quarter-mile stretch that felt like a mile as I ran.

As I crossed under the banner and the timing clock, a feeling of euphoria swept over me. After two years of blood tests, bone marrow biopsies, worrying about clinical tests, a trip to the MD Anderson Cancer Center, being told not to run, and battling depression, I had just finished my first marathon with leukemia.

My time was 4:35, and my passion was alive and well. For four and a half hours, I hurt more than I have ever experienced. Still, I had found the courage to persevere and defeat leukemia, a daunting adversary. Yet, I was not oblivious to the fact that the war had only begun. Leukemia was not going away.

As I walked toward the volunteer who was handing out the finisher medals, a thought about MD Anderson surfaced. I remembered the oncologist at MD Anderson saying, "Your energy level will become so low that you will find it difficult just taking out the trash." I chuckled under my breath as I reflected, *He was definitely correct about that, especially when the trash bin is 26.2 miles away.*

As I collected my finisher's medal, the runner who spoke to me during the incline tapped my shoulder. After our encounter, I had never watched to see if he passed me or if he was still behind me. My focus was on trying to finish.

"Thanks for dragging me to the finish. I don't think I would have made it without you to follow."

I laughed, responding, "'Dragging' is certainly the way I would describe my finish."

My accomplishment now felt even better.

I knew Will would finish ahead of me and wait for Don, but I did not see him. I was too fatigued to be able to focus, so I started walking (actually, staggering) back to the hotel. As I finished showering, Will and Don arrived. Will handed me a mug that had "Age Group Award" painted on the side. I had finished second in my age group. *Unbelievable,* I thought. *Before leukemia, I had never placed in the top three in my age group at any road race.*

Don and Will showered and drove back to Mobile. I crawled into bed for an afternoon of sleep and relaxation. I lay there reflecting on the day's event. In spite of the oncologist's warnings, I had just completed 26.2 miles without any life-threatening consequences. Yes, there was an unpleasant introduction to a new level of suffering, and I had wanted to stop several times. Yet, I pushed myself well beyond my perceived pain threshold, and I had never before felt more alive. In addition, I had helped someone else finish.

My final thoughts before falling asleep were, *My finishing time was only thirty-five minutes short of qualifying for Boston. For now, the road back to Boston does not look so long.*

CHAPTER 21

Developing a Goal

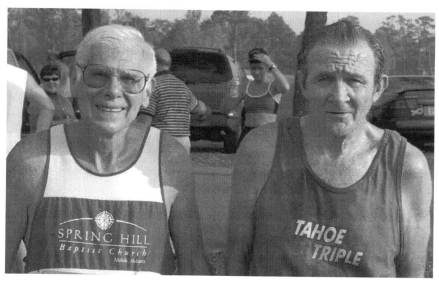

Left to Right: Will Wright and Don Withers (2004)

The greater danger for most of us lies
not setting our aim too high and falling short;
but in setting our aim too low, and achieving our mark.

Michelangelo[23]

The week following the Pensacola Marathon, I experienced a new feeling. The best way I can describe it is what I understand a drug addict experiences during withdrawal. Running the Pensacola

Marathon freed me from thoughts about leukemia and stimulated some unused cranial neurons. Now, I needed a fix to satisfy them. I needed to run another marathon, and soon.

Will and Don were going to run the Little Rock Marathon in Arkansas the following month (March 15, 2009). They invited me to join them and share their room. Needing that fix I thought, *What the heck. Why not?*

I was now on my way to becoming a marathon junkie. I was no longer Leukemia Patient #737908. I was Phillip Fields, marathon runner who happened to have leukemia.

We arrived in Little Rock the day before the marathon, checked into the hotel, and headed to the runners' expo to pick up our race packets. There was a booth manned by an organization called Marathon Maniacs.

"Don, what is a Marathon Maniac?" I inquired.

"They are a bizarre bunch of runners who do very crazy things when it comes to running marathons. The club has varying levels of entry into membership that require weird accomplishments," he replied, seeming to brush off the group.

"Like what?" I asked.

"Like running three marathons in three days," Don answered.

"So, you and Will are members? After all, you ran the Lake Tahoe triple," I reminded him.

"No. We never joined. That bunch is too weird for us. We would not fit in."

"Yeah, right," I muttered as I laughed. Don joined in the laughter. It would be several years before I thought about the Marathon Maniacs again.

We visited a booth manned by people working for Marathon Tours. Don and Will talked to them about the Athens Marathon in Greece. They put their names on a list for the 2011 trip, where Don would run his 200th marathon. What a way to celebrate his accomplishment: the site of the first marathon.

• • •

The original marathon was in 490 BC. Persia was preparing to conquer Athens. A Greek runner, Pheidippides, ran 140 miles over mountainous terrain to Sparta to solicit their help. He then ran 140 miles back to Athens, 25 miles to the Plains of Marathon, and fought the Persians. After the Battle of Marathon, Pheidippides ran the 25 miles from the battlefield at Marathon to Athens in order to relay news of the victory. He only said, "Niki! Niki!" (Victory! Victory!) "Nenikekamen!" (Rejoice! We were victorious!) He then collapsed and died from exhaustion. (This last part of the story is supposedly a legend. Others report that a different runner ran from Marathon to Athens.)

Either way, that run became the inspiration for the modern-day marathon, introduced at the 1896 modern Olympics in Athens, Greece. The distance for the marathon at that Olympics was 24.85 miles. In 1908, they increased the distance to 26.2 miles so that the marathon, which began at Windsor Castle, could finish in front of King Edward VII's royal box at White City Stadium in London. Running a marathon with leukemia, I wish the distance were still 24.85 miles.

• • •

Athens would also be Don's last marathon. Why? Don Withers had Parkinson's disease. Over the years, I watched him go from qualifying and running the Boston Marathon to completing a marathon with hiking poles. This really puts my struggle into perspective. Whenever I begin to feel sorry for myself, I think of Don. His running shoes were definitely worse than mine were.

After getting our race packets, we went to the premarathon pasta dinner that the race authorities had organized. While eating spaghetti, I heard more stories of Will and Don's marathon travels. I heard about places that I had always wanted to visit. A marathon would certainly be a good excuse to do so. I also learned about the website marathonguide.com that lists, by date, every marathon in the world. I did not know it, but everything was beginning to fall into place for my future goal.

Back at the hotel room, we laid out our marathon gear for the morning race, climbed into bed, and turned out the lights for an evening of sleep. Before falling asleep, my thoughts drifted to the stories that Will and Don had shared earlier that day. Their story of running a marathon in each of the fifty states intrigued me. This would be a way to meet my newfound need to run marathons, and to sightsee across the country at the same time. It seemed like a no-brainer and I decided that evening that I would become a member of the 50 States Marathon Club. I began formulating a game plan for my goal.

First, there would be limits placed on the goal. I would complete a marathon in all fifty states and in Washington, DC by December 2012. (That would be fifty-one marathons in forty-seven months) Why December 2012? It was now March 2009, sixteen months since my leukemia diagnosis (November 2007). December 2012 would be five years since my diagnosis and six years since my first symptoms appeared (December 2006). If I truly had only five to seven years left to live, I could not afford to drag this goal out over ten to twelve years.

Second, I would not count states in this tally in which I had run before my leukemia diagnosis; I would run all fifty states anew. This was part of my personal challenge—no shortcuts and no self-pity in my attempt to feel normal.

My next thought was, *How will I train if I am going to run one and sometimes two marathons a month?* After pondering that issue, I concluded that it would depend on how many weeks I had between marathons. During the week, I would run my usual five to six miles each day and run half-mile and mile repeats on Wednesdays. The weekend after a marathon and the weekend before a marathon, my long run would be only ten miles. If I had an additional weekend between marathons, I would run fifteen miles. I reasoned, *Running all of these marathons will help me reach my ultimate goal of again qualifying for the Boston Marathon.*

My concentration was suddenly broken when the bathroom light came on. Don began fumbling around in the half-dark bedroom and putting on his running gear. Confused, I thought, *Surely, it cannot be time to get up for the marathon.*

Will and Don were going to catch a flight back to Mobile right after the marathon. Because of his Parkinson's, Don had opted for an early start. He would begin at 7 a.m. rather than at the normal 8 a.m. I rolled over and looked at the clock.

"Don, what are you doing up? It is only half past two. The early start is not for another four and one-half hours."

"I could not sleep and decided to get up and get dressed," he answered.

"Don, reset the alarm and go back to bed," Will responded.

Don did as instructed.

When the alarm sounded, I contemplated going back to sleep and skipping the marathon. My mind and body were again competing with each other. *Do I continue with this goal or go back to sleep?*

A while later, the gun signaled the start of my second marathon in as many months. Leukemia had again taken a back seat in my mind, and a Timex Ironman watch had replaced my hourglass of life.

I previously mentioned that expending all my energy and leaving nothing on the course during a race is part of the thrill of running a marathon. However, throughout this race, I found myself doubled over, leaving something extra on the course. During one of these stops, I wondered if this new goal would be more than I could chew, or at least more than I could keep down. I was not sure why I was throwing up. It was not because of anything I had eaten. Maybe my gastrointestinal tract was reacting to anoxia created by my low red blood cell count. Maybe it was a vagal nerve response to the stress I was exposing my body to by running with leukemia. Whatever the reason, this unpleasant occurrence would become a common event during most of my future marathons.

At mile 18, I caught up to Don, who had made the early start. He was struggling to finish, as was I. We briefly spoke and shared words of encouragement. I thought to myself, *If Don can do this with Parkinson's, I can surely do it with leukemia.*

I finished at 4:48. Don also finished, and he and Will showered and rushed to the airport to catch their flight back to Mobile. I conducted what would become my usual postmarathon ritual: showering and lying in bed, relaxing for the rest of the afternoon.

As I lay in bed, many thoughts raced through my head. After running in just two marathons, it was obvious that my fifty-state goal was going to be a grueling undertaking. I wondered, *What will running marathons with leukemia eventually do to me? Will I experience hemorrhaging and a ruptured spleen like the oncologist warned?* I concluded that I would deal with those issues when they occurred. For now, I was fighting for what I loved. I was fighting to maintain my identity—a marathon runner.

The fatigue and physical toll that running marathons took on my body were only two of the many hurdles I contemplated while lying in bed. Scheduling one and sometimes two marathons each month around my yearlong teaching job would be a challenge. I do not like traveling all day on the day before a marathon. In addition, I am too fatigued to catch a flight immediately after a marathon. Thus, I would need a day to travel to a marathon, a day for the packet pickup and sightseeing, a day for the marathon, and a day to fly back home. Consequently, I would need two vacation days per marathon to make my schedule work.

If something special were near, like a national park, I would need to find a marathon near the park when I had a full week without teaching responsibilities.

Another consideration was the time of year in which to schedule a particular marathon. Because of the heat, I would need to save northern states for the summer months and southern states for the winter months.

At the time, vacation time was not a problem. I had not used many days over my previous twenty-five years of employment. I had accumulated forty-five days of vacation time, and I receive an additional two days each month. I did not want to contemplate what I would do if I got injured or required chemotherapy. It is difficult to develop a backup plan for the unknown. If either occurred, I would just have to be creative.

I did not want to focus on the four years that it would take me to reach my fifty-state goal. Whenever I start a project, I do not like to drag out its completion. Four years seemed like a long time to me. If I were to dwell on that, it might discourage me. I do not remember where, but I read, "Don't think about the mountain—just climb." I was now climbing.

I would never have considered attempting such an undertaking before my leukemia diagnosis. It sounded insane. Of course, before 2007, no one told me my average life expectancy with leukemia would be five to seven years. "Insane" seemed like the best alternative for my remaining years.

When you stop and think about it, none of us knows when our lives will end. Unless a catastrophic illness befalls us, we never think about dying. At least I didn't. Consequently, I never properly prepared for dying. Now, in a way, I was fortunate. Because of my diagnosis, I had begun to live as if each day was my last. Here is a bit of advice: Do not wait for an unfavorable diagnosis before you get things in order or get right with God.

For now, I had a purpose to keep me moving forward. This goal allowed me to feel normal and to feel alive in spite of leukemia. I would visualize leukemia as nothing more than another trip, but a trip I would use to my advantage. This blood cancer would be my motivation to travel to places I had always wanted to see. Before, I had excuses not to do so—things like work, money, or time. Now, time was the real enemy, and the word *procrastination* was no longer in my vocabulary. I could no longer place my dreams on the back burner. For me, the time was and always will be now.

If you have been dreaming about doing something, do not delay any longer. We sometimes sing a hymn at mass entitled *Eye Has Not Seen*. It says, "Our lives are but a single breath, we flower and we fade." Now, I no longer miss an opportunity to visit my family. Whenever possible, I say, "I love you," "I am sorry," "I forgive you," and "thank you." When it is time, if I am able, I will say, "Goodbye." Until then, I still have lots of living, laughing, and loving to do.

CHAPTER 22
Developing an Attitude

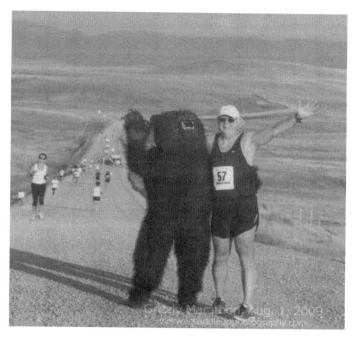

Grizzly Marathon, Montana (2009)

*Don't let the pain of one season
destroy the joy of all the rest.*

Anonymous

After returning from Arkansas, I ran an 8K race in Mobile, Alabama. There, I overheard a runner, Marian Loftin, talking about going to Louisville, Kentucky, to visit her family and to run the Kentucky Derby Festival Marathon on April 15, 2009. Since there would be someone I knew at the race, I registered for my third marathon in as many months.

This would be among my five worst marathons, and it would be the hottest. By mile 5, the water at the aid stations was too warm to drink. At mile 6, the shadow I was casting to my right was entertaining me. I looked for anything during that marathon that would provide a diversion from the pain. Later, a second shadow appeared on my left, and I thought a runner was getting ready to pass me. However, the runner did not go by, and the shadow lingered. I glanced over my left shoulder to see who it was. No one was there. I was casting a second shadow to my left as well.

I thought, *Wow*! *Two shadows, is that possible*? I wondered if I was hallucinating because of the heat. Maybe it was the Angel of Death running beside me. If it was, he must have found someone in worse shape than me because he disappeared.

Here is a question for all of you marathon runners: Do you keep seeing the same person throughout a marathon? While in a port-o-let line at the start of the Kentucky Derby Festival Marathon, I saw a woman in a strange outfit: a pink tutu and pink antennae on her head—not an outfit you could easily forget. I again saw her at the starting line standing directly behind me. This time she waved to me. During the marathon, when I turned to see who was casting that shadow on my left, I was expecting to see the pink antennae.

While approaching the finish line, I had a sensation that someone was staring at me. I did not want to look, but I eventually did. There, in the spectator bleachers, was the woman with the pink antennae. Again, she waved to me, causing me to trip over my own feet and almost fall.

While sitting in a chair in the finish area, I thought, *Did I really see that woman in the bleachers? Was she an illusion? Surely, the Angel of Death would not wear such a costume.* Nevertheless, I discreetly pinched myself to see if I was alive.

My finish time was 5:34. This was my first ever five-hour marathon. It would not be my last. I added heat to my list of things that increased the stress of cancer-related fatigue.

Marian invited me to join her and her family for dinner that evening. During the meal, Marian expressed a desire to run a marathon in all fifty states, not realizing that I had the same goal. That evening, we made a pact to train and pursue the goal together. From now on in this book, when you see the word *we*, I am referring to Marian and me.

The Green Bay Marathon in Wisconsin on May 17, 2009, was my fourth marathon with leukemia. Near the finish line, we ran into Lambeau Field, the Green Bay Packers' football stadium. As I circled the track, I could see myself on the JumboTron. Music was blaring from speakers in the stadium. The seats on the exit side of the stadium were full of spectators cheering the runners. When I reached that side of the stadium, *Twist and Shout* was blaring from the speakers. I stopped in front of the crowd and did the Twist.

The crowd cheered loudly at my ridiculous-looking dance contortions. They did not realize I was doing my "dance" because of the cramping in nearly every muscle in my body. I quickly exited the stadium before I fell down and made an even bigger fool of myself. I crossed the finish line in 4:40.

I found a chair in the shade to sit on and throw up while Marian went to the food tent for a bratwurst sandwich and beer (**Chapter Related Memory: Bratwurst.** The story is at the end of the chapter).

My next marathon was the Estes Park Marathon in Colorado on June 14, 2009. The highlight of the trip was the sightseeing before the marathon. It was 14,000 feet to the top of the snow-covered tundra, and the view was spectacular. At the lower elevations, there were moose, elk, and fat marmots.

Like Louisville, the Estes Park Marathon was among my five worst marathons. Because of my low red blood cell count and coming down with the flu just days before the marathon, the 7,500-foot altitude created a significant hurdle. I added high altitude to the list (heat and hills) of marathon obstacles that my leukemia would exacerbate.

I remember one aid station in particular that was located within the last ten miles. A volunteer had a tub of towels soaking in ice water. I stood there for a long time with one of those towels around my neck. While enjoying the welcomed relief, I focused on the snow-covered Rocky Mountains in the distance. As I replaced the towel in the ice bath, the volunteer said, "You are welcome to keep it."

I declined, saying, "Runners behind me might need it more."

She looked at me sort of funny and said, "I don't think so."

I wondered, *Do I look that bad, or am I the last runner?*

I crossed the finish line in 6:04 and lay on a bench in the shade. I watched as other runners completed the marathon. I chuckled to myself, thinking, *I did not finish last. Therefore, I just must have looked bad to the volunteer handing out the towels.*

The Grandfather Mountain Marathon on July 11, 2009, would be my hilliest marathon. It was twenty-four miles up a switchback road to the top of Grandfather Mountain. I made it to the top in 5:05. It was a hard battle because of my cancer-related fatigue, but I had won. There would be many more such battles to fight in this war with leukemia, but I was slowly developing an ally to assist me—an attitude. After all, leukemia had not shown me anything yet to stop me from reaching my goal.

There is a quote by Brian Tracy: "You cannot control what happens to you, but you can control your attitude toward what happens to you. And in that, you will be mastering change rather than allowing it to master you."[24]

I was only beginning to learn how to control my attitude toward having leukemia. My biggest challenge was not to let my negative feelings affect those around me. When one feels awful all the time, it takes a lot of effort not to complain. I worried, *If I complain, soon everyone will hate seeing me approach.*

After the marathon, we took the bus back down the mountain to our car at the starting line. There was a woman on the bus who had apparently suffered a vascular insult running up that mountain and had lost her vision. It seems like I am constantly crossing paths with someone with whom I would not trade my running shoes. These encounters remind me that the poker hand dealt to us is not always the one we choose. What is important is what we do with the hand we are dealt. We can fold or continue playing in hopes that things will improve.

The Grizzly Marathon in Choteau, Montana, on August 1, 2009 was marathon number seven in seven months. Montana is appropriately nicknamed Big Sky Country. During the marathon, there was only bright blue sky and wheat fields that stretched as far as I could see. In the distance, the wheat and sky merged. My finish time was 5:44.

Marian and I spent the next three days hiking in Glacier National Park where the wildlife was bountiful. On one trail, a family of mountain goats, traveling in the opposite direction, approached us. They appeared to be playing chicken, unwilling to cede the pathway to us; we relented. They meandered past us within touching distance (though we did not touch them—their sharp, pointed horns were an enormous deterrent from getting too friendly). Bighorn sheep, deer, and marmots were ever-present in the meadows.

The most exciting hike in the park was one led by a park ranger to Grinnell Glacier. It was a six-mile and four-hour climb to the glacier. On the way up, the ranger told us about the history of the park glaciers. We also learned about the park flora and wildlife.

The trail went through berry-covered mountainsides, feeding grounds of brown bears. We were encouraged to stay together as a group; that way, we would look bigger than any bear. There was another advantage to doing the hike with a group rather than going alone: If a bear attacks, you only have to be faster than one other person is.

My finish time at the New Mexico Marathon in Albuquerque on September 6, 2009 was 5:14. During the marathon, hot air balloons lifted off the ground and filled the sky with their colorful bags. I had to be careful where I planted my feet while running. Tarantula spiders were warming themselves on the road.

On October 4, I traveled with Will Wright to the Wineglass Marathon in Corning, New York. We took a bus to the start of the marathon in Bath, New York, which has numerous wineries, and we finished in Corning, New York, which is the home of the

Corning Glass factory. Hence, the marathon name, "Wineglass." I was excited about finishing the marathon in 4:33. It had been a long time since I had run a marathon in less than five hours, and I had begun to think that leukemia was winning the race through the fifty states. I now thought, *Not so fast, you filthy blood cancer. I still have some fight left in me.*

The Marshall University Marathon in Huntington, West Virginia, on November 1, 2009 was marathon number 10 in as many months. Fall leaves and Halloween pumpkins decorated the landscape. This combination created a serene backdrop for the marathon. This tranquility also served as a memorial for a 1970 airline tragedy. A Southern Airways charter flight had crashed into a rainy hillside in Wayne County, West Virginia. Seventy-five people had died in the crash, including most of the Marshall University football team (the Thundering Herd), coaches, flight crew, and numerous fans. This was the worst single air tragedy in the history of the National Collegiate Athletic Association.

The marathon finished inside the Joan C. Edwards stadium. Volunteers tossed each runner a football as we approached the finish line. Spectators booed if any of us dropped the pass; they cheered me.

This was my second consecutive marathon with a finishing time of 4:32. Now I felt pumped. Just maybe Boston was a possibility.

Marathon number 11 in 2009 was the Kiawah Island Marathon (December 12) in South Carolina. My time was 4:43. The day after the marathon, Marian and I drove to Charleston, South Carolina. We took a tour of the historic district with its beautiful old mansions and Battery Park, sight of the first shot fired during the Civil War on April 12, 1861.

Leukemia was extracting enormous physical energy from me, and each marathon was taking me to a new level of tolerance for discomfort. Heat, humidity, hills, and high altitude had become my four horses of the apocalypse—the biblical ones. With each marathon, I had to dig deeper into my kiai just to finish. I hoped I did not have to dig much deeper. My shovel was getting dull.

I was beginning to feel like Don Quixote, jousting with windmills, his imaginary dragons. My windmills were marathons; my dragon, leukemia, was real.

I was beginning to agree with the oncologist at MD Anderson who had said that running marathons and leukemia are not compatible. I was starting to doubt my ability to maintain my monthly schedule. Yet, I had now become a marathon addict, and I did not have any desire to stop running. After all, marathons and travel provided an outlet from worries about leukemia. I continued down that road.

I enjoy reading the poem by Robert Frost titled "The Road Not Taken." It speaks of a path that diverges in a wood, and taking the one less traveled made all the difference. The road I chose has made all the difference. I was doing what I loved, running marathons. In addition, I was seeing the country and creating many great memories.

Importantly, I made it through another year without requiring chemotherapy. In January 2008, the oncologist at MD Anderson had told me that it would likely begin in three months. Being wrong about that, maybe he was wrong about the five-to-seven years. For now, though, I told myself, *I will trust in God and stay on my schedule of one marathon per month.*

Having completed eleven of fifty marathons, I looked forward to my 2010 marathon calendar. There would be new places to visit and more memories to take home with me. Thanks to leukemia, I was beginning to see all of God's wonderful creations.

Chapter Related Memory: Bratwurst

I found a chair in the shade to sit on and throw up while Marian went to the food tent for a bratwurst sandwich and beer.

The summer after my fifth grade, Mom put me on a train with a suitcase and a bag of sandwiches. My destination was Defiance, Ohio, and a fun-filled summer with my four aunts.

To a ten-year-boy, riding a train was a big thrill. There was so much to see and fantasize about; I was a U.S. Marshal riding guard on a train that was carrying the payroll to the miners, or I was a soldier helping to protect the train from Indians. I thought, *Boy, oh boy! When the sixth grade starts up in the fall, I will have such a story to tell my classmates!*

While staying with Aunt Sophia, I heard someone rummaging around in the kitchen early one morning. Going downstairs to investigate, I found Uncle Earl sitting down to a breakfast of bratwurst, sauerkraut, and beer. The rest of my visit with them included an early morning breakfast with Uncle Earl, which was always the same. (I omitted the beer from the tales I related to my classmates.)

CHAPTER 23
A Sense of Urgency

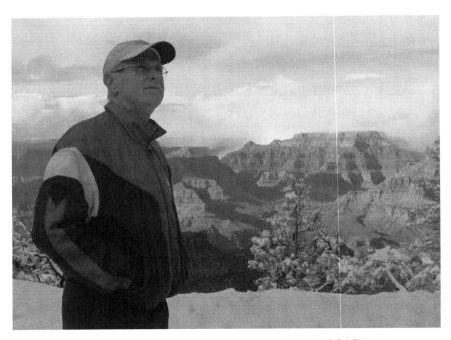

South Rim Trail, Grand Canyon (2010)

Life is not measured by the number of breaths we take,
but by the moments that take our breath away.
Vicki Corona[25]

As a new year (2010) began, my white blood cell count continued
to increase. Fortunately, it had not begun doubling, and there was

no discussion about chemotherapy. Although, like a time bomb with no clock, I knew it would eventually go off—just not when. I was glad that I had marathons and travel to focus on.

I began the year with the Mississippi Blues Marathon in Jackson, Mississippi, on January 9—the coldest marathon I would run. It was ten degrees at the start. Cold temperatures like this are now my ideal running weather. This was probably the reason for my 4:25 finishing time.

The Sedona, Arizona Marathon on February 6, 2010 was a beautiful out-and-back course through red sandstone mountains. My finishing time was a slow 5:20, and I never did get the red color out of my running shoes.

The Sedona Marathon was warm enough for running shorts and a singlet—it was snowing the next morning. Marian and I packed and drove to the south rim of the Grand Canyon.

The first part of the trip was over the breathtakingly beautiful ice- and snow-blanketed Oak Creek Canyon Road. Dense clouds blocked the sun from our view. This, coupled with everything covered with ice and snow, created a surreal backdrop. The landscape appeared pastel blue, and I felt like we had crossed over into *The Twilight Zone*. The only thing missing was Serling's voice; "You're traveling through another dimension, a dimension not only of sight and sound but of mind. A journey into a wondrous land whose boundaries are that of imagination. That's the signpost up ahead - your next stop, the Twilight Zone!" Thankfully, the signpost I read was Highway 64, and our next stop was the Grand Canyon.

There are certain things that you should do when visiting a national park. First, book a room at the main park lodge in order to get the full experience. Many are historical and have a wonderful ambiance, and they are conveniently located for sightseeing. At the Grand Canyon, we stayed at El Tovar.

Next, go to the Visitor's Center and watch the movie about the park. Lastly, check the schedule of ranger-led hikes and talks, and participate in as many of them as your visit will allow. By doing all this, you will learn how the landscape formed millions of years ago, the history of the ancient people who migrated through the area, and the ecological balance between the animals and the land.

We learned that the Grand Canyon is part of the Colorado Plateau that began to rise 60 million years ago. This Plateau covers part of Colorado, Utah, Arizona, and New Mexico.

When we arrived, it was snowing and the fog was so thick that the Canyon was not visible. The next morning, the fog cleared, and we had a panoramic view of an amazing landscape.

Deep snow covered the twelve miles of the Canyon Rim hiking trail. While we were hiking the trail, the only sounds we heard were those of the snow crunching under our feet and ravens croaking in the distance. A flock of them seemed to be playing a game at the rim. They dipped and dove into the canyon, only to soon reappear like missiles shot from the canyon floor.

The views from the trail were breathtaking. Each evening, the sunset reflected over the snow-covered face of Maricopa Point next to El Tovar. Viewing the moon and the stars above the Grand Canyon was a spectacular sight. Hopi Point was a great canyon overlook to watch the beautiful orange and purple hues of the sunrise. I felt blessed that leukemia had brought me there in the morning. While looking out over the canyon, I marveled at God's creation.

We left the Grand Canyon and visited the Painted Desert and the Petrified Forest. In grade school, I dreamed of becoming an archeologist. At bedtime, Mom would read stories to me about the Petrified Forest. During the late Triassic Period, over 225 million years ago, Arizona was part of the largest global landmass, Pangaea. This region was a tropical environment. Trees felled by wind, erosion, or death by insects ended up in the waterways and were buried in the mud for millions of years. Over time, wind erosion uncovered what is now the Petrified Forest. There is still more yet to be unearthed. There is no wood in the Petrified Forest. Minerals like iron, pyrite, manganese dioxide, silica, and goethite replaced it. They call the process "permineralization," and it gives the fossilized logs their brilliant colors. Although the logs appear as if someone sawed them into pieces, they actually fractured over time.

Now, so many years after hearing stories about the Petrified Forest, I was walking among those trees. Running in the fifty states had brought to life one of my childhood dreams. Mom had died a little over five years earlier, and I was saddened that she was not sharing my dreams. Yet, who knows? Maybe she was.

Next on my schedule was the Snickers Energy Bar Marathon in Albany, Georgia, on March 6, 2010. This was the first marathon I would run with a pacer. These runners pace other runners to a three to five hour finish. This pacer was pacing runners to a 4:30 finish, running with a Garmin watch and maintaining a steady pace the whole way. My finishing time was 4:35. That is when I decided, *I am getting one of those watches when I get home.*

The preferred transportation to and from the National Marathon in Washington, DC, on March 20, 2010 was the subway. There was a long and steep escalator out of the subway tunnel. It was working on the way to the marathon but not on the way back. After the marathon, it was humorous watching almost everyone walking down the escalator backwards. I had often wondered if that form of postmarathon stair travel was unique to me. Now I know.

The Charlottesville Marathon in Virginia on April 20, 2010 began with a mildly hilly out-and-back first half. This part of the course was along a country road with a display of horse farms. We ran past lush green pastures surrounded by white wooden fences. The morning smells of wet grass and fresh horse manure were refreshing.

The hills on the initial loop were only a warm-up of things to come. The second half was a double loop of extreme hills through town. They say that the repetition of a mantra can induce a trance-like state that leads the participant to a higher level of spiritual awareness. I tested that theory; my repetition of the phrase "Hills are my friends" only served to deprive me of much needed oxygen. The only awareness I reached was that of my spirit departing from me. I finished in 4:51.

The day after the marathon, Marian and I visited Monticello, the home of Thomas Jefferson, our third president and author of the Declaration of Independence.

The marathon I ran with the most unusual name and history was The Flying Pig Marathon in Cincinnati, Ohio, on May 2, 2010. The marathon course crossed the Ohio River into Kentucky and then back into Ohio. Several bridges across the Ohio River are colorfully painted. One bridge is purple, and they call it the Purple People Bridge. Running over that bridge brought back memories of the ninth grade and a talent show. Wanda Moore, a friend of Mom, played the guitar, and I sang *Purple People Eater*. The song is about a strange creature that descends to earth because it wants to be in a rock 'n' roll band. Sheb Wooley wrote and sang the song.

As Wanda began strumming her guitar, I stood center stage, ready to sing. The audience contained students from the ninth through twelfth grades and their parents. Suddenly, I thought, *Oh, crap. I cannot remember how the song begins.* Wanda restarted the music several times, watching me carefully, but I stood silent and still. Fear had taken over, and my mind had shut down completely.

Jackie Huggins and his friends were sitting on the front row. They began booing and throwing paper balls at me. Being hit in the face by one of their missiles shocked me back to reality and I began singing.

Along the Ohio River is the beautifully manicured Friendship/Riverfront Park. Statues of pigs rest atop steam-boat-stacks at one of the entrances into Friendship Park. It is a strange emblem for a city, although like most oddities, it has a colorful history. In the early nineteenth century, critics called Cincinnati "Porkopolis," making fun of this frontier city and its meatpacking industry, which some folks around the country found distasteful. Entrepreneurial citizens welded wings to the pigs atop the steamboat-stacks. Cincinnati turned the disparaging label into a symbol of civic pride and named the marathon after that symbol (**Chapter Related Memory: Pork Chop.** The story is at the end of the chapter). My finishing time was 4:48.

On May 30, 2010, I finished the Vermont City Marathon in 4:45. After the marathon, Marian and I took a cruise around Lake Champlain aboard *Spirit of Ethan Allen III*. Although we did not see the lake's friendly sea monster, "Champ," we enjoyed a steak dinner aboard the vessel.

The next three marathons I traveled alone and did not do any sightseeing. I completed Grandma's Marathon in Duluth,

Minnesota, on June 19, 2010, in 4:59; the Carrollton Festival of Races Marathon in Carrollton, Michigan, on July 25, 2010 in 5:12; and The Erie Marathon in Pennsylvania on September 12, 2010 in 4:56.

The Run Crazy Horse Marathon on October 3, 2010 was in the Black Hills and Badlands of South Dakota. This was the first of three consecutive months in which we ran marathons on back-to-back weekends. The marathon began at the Crazy Horse Memorial and went along an old railroad grade of finely crushed gravel, the Mickelson Trail. A canopy of trees covered the trails and provided shade for most of the run. The fall foliage, mixed with that of the white bark of the birch trees, was a spectacular backdrop for this marathon.

The elevation was 6,500 feet, and at one point in the run, I had trouble breathing—probably because of my low red blood cell count. While leaning against an old wooden rail fence, I was hoping this would not be a DNF. (In this case, "deceased not finished" instead of "did not finish.") Soon I was able to begin walking and then an easy jog. I had become accustomed to this occurring whenever elevation or hills were a feature of a marathon. Still, not knowing when it would occur made me uneasy as I continually waited for it to hit. It is like running under a dark rain cloud and wondering if a lightning bolt is going to strike you.

In the last six miles, a group of us battled for last place. I eventually outdistanced them and crossed the finish line in 5:59. I was first in my age group. Of course, I was the only one in my age group (60-65). I was 63 years old.

The day after the marathon, Marian and I drove to Mount Rushmore with its carvings of Washington, Jefferson, Lincoln, and Theodore Roosevelt.

I finished the Prairie Fire Marathon in Wichita, Kansas, in 5:17. This marathon would have the most unusual date; October 10, 2010 (10/10/10). That was not the only odd occurrence. (That story is for the next chapter.)

Upon returning to Mobile from the Prairie Fire Marathon, I went for my monthly blood sampling. The results were not good. The quality of my blood had deteriorated more rapidly than during the previous two months. To this day, I remember sitting in the examination room and Dr. Butler saying, "You need to start mentally preparing yourself for chemotherapy." This was the last thing I had expected to hear. Because of my marathon travels, chemotherapy had become a distant speck in the recesses of my mind. I had grown accustomed to my new companion, leukemia, and I figured that we would continue to enjoy our carefree journey until I completed my goal. Now, my marathon schedule developed a sense of urgency. With chemotherapy lurking, I felt that the marathons were not occurring fast enough.

I completed the Manchester Marathon on November 7, 2010 in New Hampshire in 5:08. The day after the marathon, Marian and I drove to Salem. There, we visited the Salem Witch Trial Memorial and walked through the old village. Most of the shops displayed witchcraft memorabilia. After lunch, we sat on a street bench and watched people who were hanging out in witch costumes. (Of course, maybe they were not in costume.)

The Pensacola Marathon on November 14, 2010 was my only repeat of a state while I had leukemia. It took me an hour longer to finish (5:35) than it had in February 2009. This time my white blood cells were several hundred thousand counts higher than in 2009.

I completed the Baton Rouge Beach Marathon on December 4, 2010 in 4:58.

A week later, we ran The Rehoboth Shore Marathon in Delaware (December 11, 2010). The race began at the edge of the Atlantic Ocean, and we ran over country roads, across marshlands, and on forest trails. At several places along the course, incessant honking from nearby Canadian geese serenaded us. The sound was something akin to taxi cab drivers honking horns in New York City. My time was 4:58.

I had been seeing runners wearing Marathon Maniac shirts. I recalled my conversation with Don Withers at the Little Rock Marathon almost two years earlier. I qualified in 2010 for membership in the club because I had completed sixteen marathons in sixteen different states in twelve months, and I joined at the Osmium level.

As 2010 ended, I had completed twenty-seven marathons and I was over halfway to my goal. My average finishing time was 5:01. As my Dad would have said, "Leukemia, take and stick that in your pipe and smoke on it."

Chapter Related Memory: Pork Chop

Entrepreneurial citizens welded wings to the pigs atop the steamboat-stacks. Cincinnati turned the disparaging label into a symbol of civic pride and named the marathon after that symbol.

When I was eight years old, my brother's pig almost ate me. His 4-H project was not your typical pot-bellied pet. She was a 400-pound sow that Michael had named Pork Chop. She was huge and outweighed me by 300 pounds. I went into the pigpen to pet Pork Chop's babies, and she chased me around her enclosure.

She grabbed me by my butt and pulled me down into the mud. Fortunately, Michael was there to help me to safety.

Pork Chop ate anything that got into her pen when she had piglets. She ate our chickens and our pet white duck named Quack-Quack. She tried to eat our pet dachshund, Trudy, and she tried to eat me.

CHAPTER 24
Melanie

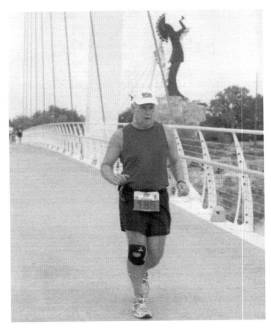

Wichita Marathon, Kansas (2010)

God did not comfort us so we would be comfortable.
He comforted us so we would be comforters.

Paraphrase of Apostle Paul (2 Corinthians 1:4)

To date, one marathon stands out from all the others. This is not because of where it was, the course, or the sightseeing afterwards.

Something happened that changed my approach to completing a marathon in all the states and shifted my goal to one that was less self-serving.

I had stuck to my one-marathon-per-month schedule, but something seemed to be missing. I did not feel good about myself. This was a troubling feeling that I had been having since Mom's death in 2004. Over the next six years, I had a constant mental itch that I could not seem to scratch. I liken it to a jingle that plays repeatedly in your subconscious and just will not go away.

Every so often, I replayed Mom's words to my brother and me: "Throughout your lives, you will be taking various trips. What you get out of these trips will be left up to you." Well, I was certainly getting a lot out of my trips. I was completing a goal and creating wonderful memories. However, that nagging feeling was always there: *What am I not doing?*

I reflected on Mom's life in Bushnell as Sumter County's first health nurse. I recalled how she reached out to the community and its people. God called her to a higher purpose—community service—and she responded.

Maybe this emotional dark cloud was a feeling that I was letting her down, that I was not doing enough for those around me. I was not following the road map she had left behind.

Sure, people told me, "You teach students! You inspire them in their profession!" Some said I was doing research that might advance reproductive health care, as though that should be enough to resolve my "reaching out" itch. None of those things did. It was as if Mom were looking down and saying, "Get off your ass and stop thinking only about your own self-fulfilling goals! Where is your stewardship?"

Mom had always been there to guide me. She had a way of conveying information in subtle ways without coming out and stating it directly. I remember how she would cleverly provide the information. Being the county nurse, she had access to all sorts of literature about sex. When I approached puberty, she would leave pamphlets on the coffee table, hoping I would read them and ask questions. Thanks to Jackie Huggins, who was two years older than I was, Mom's information was several years too late. I would have been spared an embarrassing moment had I learned from Mom instead of Jackie (**Chapter Related Memory: The Question.** The story is at the end of the chapter).

In high school, newspaper clippings began to appear around the house, detailing the negative consequences of smoking and of drinking alcohol. When I was in college, mail from Mother contained newspaper articles about the evil, marijuana.

Now, I did not have Mom's guidance. There were no pamphlets or newspaper clippings left out for me to read. This uncomfortable feeling persisted, and I was unsure what to do.

As a Christian, I believe things happen for a reason. Situations can open our eyes and provide us direction, sort of like a guardian angel that God has sent to fill a missing parent's role. Maybe the angel is actually a parent. Of course, when this happens, seize the moment. Else, the opportunity will pass us by and we will continue to be lost. My moment came at the Prairie Fire Marathon in Wichita, Kansas, in October 2010. Maybe the date 10/10/10 was an omen.

The Prairie Fire Marathon race director learned about my leukemia and my goal from the registration form. He contacted me and asked if the local newspaper could interview me by phone for a human-interest piece leading up to the marathon. I had mixed feelings about doing so. For nearly three years, only my close friends knew that I had leukemia. Since no one in Kansas knew me and since the newspaper article was not likely to show up in Mobile, I agreed. It was just a straightforward article about my goal and progress thus far. I was unaware that this article would spark exactly what I needed.

I had just checked into the hotel room in Wichita when the phone rang. I answered, and a woman, living in Wichita, introduced herself as Melanie. I inquired, "How did you know where I was staying?" She responded, "I assumed that you would be staying at the marathon host hotel and wanted to reach out to you." She said that she had read the newspaper story and that what I had been able to accomplish inspired her. Doctors had recently diagnosed her young daughter with leukemia, and she was beginning chemotherapy. Until she read my story, everything had seemed hopeless. My story encouraged her and gave her family hope.

Melanie's story really touched me. When I got off the phone, I knew exactly what I had to do to fill the emptiness that I had been feeling.

I never thought to ask Melanie her last name, so she will never know how important a messenger angel she had been. I wonder if Mom sent her. Maybe this was one of Mom's pamphlets in a different form.

When I returned to Mobile, I began to research foundations that focused on research and treatment of pediatric cancer. Through a friend, I learned about the Nemours Foundation. Through his will, Alfred I. Du Pont established the Alfred I. Du Pont Testamentary Trust in 1936. He left specific instructions to create a charitable organization, which would be devoted to providing health care services to children. He named it the Nemours Foundation, after his family's homeland in France. Delivery on Du Pont's vision began in 1940 when the Alfred I. DuPont

Institute, a pediatric hospital in Wilmington, Delaware, opened its doors.

Nemours provides an integrated medical system that includes hospital- and clinic-based specialty treatment spanning primary care, prevention, research, and medical education designed to improve children's lives. It also provides social support for both the children and their families. Therefore, they address both psychosocial and emotional needs.

A friend at work, Joanne Brookfield, helped me develop a website, runningwithleukemia.org. The website went online in January 2011. The website has a link so that people can send a donation directly to Nemours for pediatric cancer patients. I had the name of my website printed on the front and back of my running shirts, as well as on the back window of my Ford F-150 truck. As of 2019, I have raised over $50,000 for pediatric oncology.

I use the website to address questions from people about exercise and the particulars of running with leukemia. I have received questions about what to expect during and after chemotherapy, and I have shared links to important publications regarding leukemia and new treatments that may soon be available. There are also photos of my travels and pages with newspaper articles about my running with leukemia. Now, I had connected my self-serving goal of running a marathon in all fifty states to a less selfish purpose: children with cancer.

The following is an e-mail I received after going online with my website:

"Dr. Fields, I'm from Jacksonville, Florida, where there is a Nemours/Wolfson Children's Hospital that I have spent a great deal of time at. I cannot speak for others, but it is a wonderful place. It was not for me, but for a younger cousin, who finally passed a few years ago at the age of 21. I spent many spring breaks and summers in there with her keeping her company when I was younger and she was 5 to 10 years old. They would do great things for the kids: bringing in clowns, the cow for some ice cream brand (cannot recall the brand, but it was Elsie the cow), silly dress-up events, and all kinds of things for the kids. They always took great care of my cousin, and I thought you might like to hear from someone who has seen firsthand how great they are."

• • •

One of my goals is to inspire others with cancer not to give up. Life does not end with a diagnosis—it only begins. I am optimistic that people will read about my journey with leukemia and continue to dream. My hope is that they, too, will live each day as if it is their last. I pray that they will spend that time in an environment that they enjoy. For example, listening to their favorite music, cherishing those they love, or watching sunrises and sunsets.

According to Albert Einstein, "There are two ways to live. You can live as if there are no miracles. Or you can live as if every day is a miracle."[26] The following is a letter about a woman who chose the latter:

"Hi, Dr. Fields, I thought about this as soon as I got off of the elevator earlier.... I just wanted to tell you thanks from a friend. I have a friend who had metastatic breast cancer. After being in remission for a few years, she found out at Christmastime that she had relapsed and it was metastatic. She was given a terrible prognosis and was really down. I forwarded her one of your e-mails and she checked out your website. She managed to get up enough resolve to choose to live anyway. She passed away this past weekend, but she was driving her own car earlier that same day. She had refused to be on hospice care and had even convinced her docs to let her participate in a trial at MD Anderson. She was supposed to leave next weekend to participate. She asked me a while back to tell you thank you. Her husband asked me again to thank you on Saturday. She will be missed terribly but because she was inspired by your website and by Nemours, her daughter won't grow up remembering her mom as sick and stuck in bed. She'll remember that her mom was planning her birthday party and always smiling, instead. So thank you from the family, and thank you from me."

• • •

Everything we know we have learned from others or we have learned through our personal experiences. It is our responsibility to pass along this information. We should all strive to be mentors. After all, we have all experienced something that will help another person. We sing a beautiful hymn at Mass entitled *Here I am Lord*. It speaks of someone who hears the voice of the Lord. The Lord says, "Who should I send? Who should I send to represent me?" And the person answers, "Here I am Lord, send me."

Chapter Related Memory: The Question

I would have been spared an embarrassing moment had I learned from Mom instead of Jackie.

I was nine years old and in the fourth grade. At lunch, I overheard a sixth-grader talking to other students about prostitutes. It was Jackie Huggins.

I asked Jackie, "What's a prostitute?"

He responded, "Oh, it's nothing important. Ask Mrs. Franklin when you get back to class."

When I returned to the classroom, I walked up to the front of the class and stood in front of Mrs. Franklin's desk. She looked up at me and smiled, "What do you want, Phillip?"

Then, loud enough for my classmates to hear, I asked, "Mrs. Franklin, what's a prostitute?" For a moment, I thought that she was going to faint. All of the color left her face, and her eyes seemed to bug out of her head. I immediately knew that I had made a mistake. However, before I could exit, she recovered her composure. "Where did you learn such a disgusting word?"

Not wanting to get Jackie in trouble I responded, "I heard some kids talking about it on the school bus. I don't know who they were."

She scribbled something on a piece of paper, pinned it to my shirt, and said, "You can just march yourself right down to the principal's office. And do not read that note."

No doubt, that note explained my transgression.

As I left the room, I could hear the snickering from my classmates. I assumed either they knew what a prostitute was or they were laughing because a teacher was punishing me—again.

The principal read the note and said, "You need to go stand in the hall for an hour and think about what you said." I immediately countered, "How can I think about what I said when I don't know what it means?"

Having not yet learned when to keep my mouth shut, I received a butt whacking with a paddle prior to standing in the hall. Back then, the paddles were like those you see designed by college fraternity members. Some teachers even drilled holes in their paddle so there was less air resistance, allowing them to obtain more velocity. This also left a funny design on my buttocks.

The paddling was less painful than standing in the hall. Being a hall statue was quite embarrassing. Anyone who walked in the hall would see me standing there and know that the principal was punishing me. I attempted to blend in with the wall, but my clothes clashed with an ugly green pastel paint. During that hour, I mused about the question, *What the heck is a prostitute?*

CHAPTER 25

It's Time

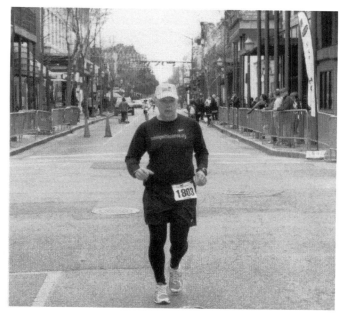

First Light Marathon, Mobile (2011)

You can't start the next chapter of your life
if you keep rereading the last one.

Unknown

In the first year of my fifty-state journey, I could run twenty-three miles of a marathon with Marian and finish less than five minutes behind her. As my white blood cell count increased, Marian was beating me by thirty, sixty, and then ninety minutes. I began to dislike going to marathons with her. She had become a barometer for my declining health.

It became painfully obvious that the way I ran marathons ten years ago, or even ten months ago, was no longer my norm. My previous accomplishments are only the way things were, memories to be looked fondly upon but left firmly in the past.

As difficult as the marathons had become, I was now satisfied with just finishing them. I thought, *Even if leukemia takes away my physical ability to run well, I will not let it take away my passion for running marathons. If I lose my passion, I lose my reason for living.* Still, there was no denying that I was getting wearier and the marathons were getting more difficult to complete. My passion had helped me through the reality and the depression of having leukemia. Yet, it was my belief in God that gave me the will to continue completing marathons with this disease fighting against me.

Whenever I felt that I could no longer run another step, I recited words from the hymn, *You Are Mine*. The song says that God is talking to me and that if I follow Him, He will bring me home. This helped carry me across the finish line, and home—again.

By the end of 2010, my total white blood cell count had begun to double between monthly blood samplings. The count had increased to over 200,000 per microliter (normal levels are 4,000 to 10,000 per microliter). The lymph nodes in my neck had become so large that I looked like a giant chipmunk stockpiling nuts for the winter. I found it hard to look in the mirror while shaving and not feel anxious. Thoughts that I could not control filled me with dread: *What does the near future have in store for me?* I kept praying, *Let me finish my goal before requiring chemotherapy.*

That was not to be. In January 2011, three years after my trip to MD Anderson, I heard those dreaded words from Dr. Butler: "It's time." Still, I viewed my glass as half-full. I had greatly exceeded the three months that Dr. Keating had originally predicted. Regardless, I questioned, "Is chemotherapy really necessary at this time?"

Dr. Butler was aware of my goal and made an appointment for me to get a second opinion at a different cancer center. He wanted me to be comfortable with his decision and with mine.

While meeting with this new oncologist, I asked the same question. "Is it really necessary that I start chemotherapy next week?"

Her response was, "You can put it off a week, maybe two, if you have things you need to do."

Nervously, I said, "I was hoping for two years. That way I can finish my goal of running a marathon in every state."

She shook her head. "Not if you want to live."

The feelings of anxiety and fear of the unknown that I experienced when I initially learned that I had leukemia resurfaced. Chemotherapy was now only a matter of scheduling.

The horror stories regarding chemotherapy were endless, and I was not sure how it would influence my running. Therefore, my next question to her was, "Can I run marathons during chemotherapy?"

She simply responded, "You won't want to."

Her words would haunt me. She had reinforced everything I had heard about chemotherapy.

Several days later, a patient counselor at the Mitchell Cancer Institute gave me a tour of the chemotherapy facility. During the visit, she led me to a room with a TV. She placed a DVD in the recorder and instructed me to watch the entire movie. Cancer patients who had gone through chemotherapy narrated the movie (although I suspect bad actors were playing the part of cancer patients). Either way, it was a rather cheesy movie.

There was a discussion about mouth sores and something called Miracle Mouthwash. The characters in the movie described a brand of toothpaste that was gentle on the gums. Next was a dialogue about precautions to take because of a lack of immunity. Topics included wearing a N95-rated facial mask when in crowds or flying, refraining from touching your face, and washing your hands regularly with soap, especially before eating. I began carrying a mask and a small bottle of hand sanitizer on my trips (**Chapter Related Memory: The Discipline Manual.** The story is at the end of the chapter).

Lastly, the people in the movie talked about hair loss. I learned that I may lose my hair, but it would come back. Of course, it might come back a different color, and it might be straight or curly. My thoughts about this were, *I find it hard to envision myself as a curly red head, although I would not mind if my hair came back with less gray in it*. Next, they demonstrated how to tie a scarf to cover a baldhead.

Good grief! I thought.

I had enough, turned the TV off, and walked out with fifteen minutes left on the movie. Later, though, I did stop at a Walgreens Pharmacy on the way home and bought the toothpaste and Miracle Mouthwash they had recommended. I guess the movie was not a complete waste of time.

After the movie, I met with Dr. Butler, and he described the chemotherapy protocol. I might require an intravenous (IV) port in my subclavian vein. (This vein is located in the upper anterior chest wall) The port would remain in place for the entire six months of chemotherapy and would be the infusion site for the chemicals.

Before my brain could completely process *infusion site for chemicals*, I heard him say, "The entry site of the port is prone to becoming infected, or it might fail after a few uses. If the latter occurs, a new one will be placed in the other subclavian vein."

The conversation created even more anxiety and depression. For six months, a port would reinforce the fact that I was not normal. In addition, the surgeon might puncture my lung during the installation of the port causing a pneumothorax (collapse of the lung). This would definitely bring a halt to my running

Dr. Butler was not yet finished with thoroughly depressing me and driving me to having nightmares. He told me I might experience nausea, fungal infections in my upper respiratory system, fatigue, and on and on. I do not remember the "on and on" since my mind had already exited the conversation.

My attention returned when I heard chemotherapy chemicals. Before I describe the compounds, let me begin by saying, if the EPA found any of these chemicals on your property, they would condemn your land as a toxic waste dump.

Dr. Butler told me that I would first receive a premedication with various drugs: ALOXI for nausea, dexamethasone for an allergic reaction and nausea, and acetaminophen for fever. In addition, there was meperidine for rigors or severe shivering, and diphenhydramine for nausea.

I replayed the mental tape of what I had just heard, *I am going to receive drugs that cause nausea, an allergic reaction, nausea, fever, rigors, and more nausea. So what about something for the depression you are causing me.*

Next, the infusion would contain rituximab, a monoclonal antibody that destroys B-cell lymphocytes. (Without B-cells, I would be susceptible to bacteria, viruses, and parasites.) The hope was that normal B-cells would develop after chemotherapy.)

After the rituximab, the nurse would attach an IV bag that would contain a special chemical cocktail. One of the chemicals would be fludarabine, which interrupts the cell cycle of dividing cells. It is most effective when cell division is greatest. This is why an oncologist waits until the white cell number is doubling in a short time period before starting chemotherapy.

Fludarabine disrupts cell division of normal cells as well, such as those of the GI tract. Of course, one of the side effects is nausea.

The other chemical would be cyclophosphamide. This compound damages cellular DNA and kills cells that are undergoing cell division. There could be potential negative reactions to this drug: nausea, hair loss, and lethargy.

Again I thought, *Lethargy! How can I possibly be more tired than I already am?* Boy, oh boy, was I in for a rude awakening. I would be wishing for the normal of the past two years.

Cyclophosphamide also affects DNA of normal cells and causes cell mutations. This could lead to adverse side effects, including heart damage, non-Hodgkin's lymphoma, kidney cancer, or bladder cancer, all of which would be more difficult to treat than the leukemia I had.

That is just dandy. I am going to possibly send my leukemia into remission and then develop an even worse medical condition, I thought.

I considered cyclophosphamide to be the Russian roulette of chemotherapy.

As if the above possible side effects of cyclophosphamide and fludarabine were not bad enough, these chemicals are myelosuppressive, which may cause hematologic toxicity. In other words, these chemicals might interfere with the ability of my bone marrow to produce new white and red blood cells. Consequently, I would remain immunocompromised and my energy level would not return to normal.

The word *normal* was becoming rather meaningless in my vocabulary. It had become a constantly changing adjective defining my ever-evolving identity.

I would receive chemotherapy over a three-day period. This would occur every twenty-one days for six treatments. Dr. Keating had recommended the same protocol.

Oncologist refer to this chemotherapy protocol as FCR (fludarabine, cyclophosphamide, and rituximab). Before I was finished with chemotherapy, I would refer to it as "SHIT."

The three days I chose for treatment were Wednesday, Thursday, and Friday at 8 a.m. I was teaching anatomy to physician assistant students at the time and did not want to impose on other faculty more than was necessary. Not being sure how I would react to the chemicals, I scheduled my lectures for Monday and Tuesday afternoons. I was hopeful that the weekend would give me sufficient time to recover from whatever side effects I might experience.

Because of my suppressed immunity, other faculty would have to teach the labs on Wednesdays, Thursdays, and Fridays. I could not chance cutting myself during a donor dissection. This could likely cause an infection that would send me to the hospital, or worse, the morgue.

An oncologist had diagnosed Dr. Lou Guillette, a friend of my brother, with CLL (chronic lymphocytic leukemia) the year before I was. He had recently gone through the FCR protocol. Therefore, I drove to Gainesville, Florida, to visit my brother and his friend. I wanted to get a sense of what was in store for me.

We sat in an enclosed patio that overlooked an alligator-infested pond surrounded by palmetto. The place was very appropriate. Lou was one of the world's authorities on the reproductive behavior and physiology of the alligator, and he had a backyard full of them.

Lou's wife graciously served us iced tea as I pulled out a sheet of paper on which I had written my list of questions. The picture Lou painted was not reassuring. I heard phrases like "indescribable nausea," "unable to eat or drink," "thought I would not survive," and "recovered from each round of treatment just in time for the next treatment."

He gave up biking because he could not chance having an accident while being immunocompromised. He did not want to end up in the emergency room with an uncontrollable infection. He praised his wife for tolerating the dreadful days and for preparing tasty and healthy meals when he was finally able to eat.

I would be on my own since I did not want to be a burden on someone—it was what I preferred.

Leaving Gainesville, I felt even less comfortable about the impending chemotherapy. I had zero assurance that I would be able to run during chemotherapy. Just like so many of my other questions on this journey, I would just have to wait and see.

I had long since changed the height on my driver's license, I had created a will and trust, and I had gone to confession. Consequently, everything was ready for what seemed like an upcoming trip to hell and back. This new journey would begin in one month. There was only one thing left to do: run a marathon.

Actually, I ran two marathons in January. The First Light Marathon (January 1, 2011) was in my hometown of Mobile, Alabama. This would be the last marathon I would finish in under five hours, coming in at 4:35. Three weeks later (January 30, 2011), I ran the Chevron Marathon in Houston, Texas. Around thirteen miles, I tore my left gastrocnemius muscle (my calf muscle) and limped to the finish line in 5:40.

The day after the marathon, Marian and I visited the Houston Holocaust Museum, which commemorates the genocide of 6 million Jews during World War II. I had recently seen a great movie called *Life is Beautiful*. The movie begins by showing the good times experienced by Jewish families in Germany. It ends with the horror these same people experienced while being systematically exterminated by the Nazi régime.

While walking through the museum it dawned on me: *I am in the hometown of MD Anderson.* This revelation open the floodgates of terrifying thoughts of what was about to happen to me. My mind was no longer free from thoughts about cancer. The impending chemotherapy that awaited me when I returned home was now the focus of my attention.

Chapter Related Memory: The Discipline Manual

Next was a dialogue about precautions to take because of a lack of immunity. Topics included carrying a N95-rated facial mask when flying, refraining from touching your face, and washing your hands regularly with soap, especially before eating.

I recall the day I chewed on a bar of soap—not intentionally! I was only five years old at the time, so my recollection of the occasion is somewhat sketchy. The incident was likely provoked because I had talked back to Mom. Before I could say, "What's in your hand?" a bar of soap was produced and scraped across my teeth. Mom must have been planning this based on one of my prior "toilet tongue" outbursts and was probably carrying the soap in her pocket. I wonder if that particular technique was in an early 1950s child psychology manual, possibly in the discipline section for a five-year-old, under the title, "How to Properly Wash Their Mouth Out with Soap."

Well, it got my attention, and I did not have to experience that punishment again. I had learned my lesson, temporarily. It was a good thing, since I am not sure I would have ever developed a taste for soap.

Discipline is a word that has a dual meaning. It can mean being in control and not letting circumstances dictate what you do. However, during my childhood, *discipline* had an entirely different meaning. In my imaginary child psychology manual from the 1950s, there was another section for eight-year-olds entitled, "Picking Out the Proper Switch." When I was eight years old, I again required an attitude adjustment. This time Mom used something other than soap. She sent me into the yard to retrieve a bough for her switch. When we moved from town to a cattle ranch, there was never a shortage of switches.

I once tried to outfox Mom and selected a rather thin branch. This only resulted in Mom picking one that was larger than usual. I was a quick learner in her classroom.

The switching apparently hurt Mom more than it hurt me; that form of punishment stopped shortly after it began. Mom, being resourceful, developed a new form of punishment. She began using a flyswatter. This did not hurt as much as the switch, but it worked much better in correcting my bad behavior. After all, imagine someone swatting you with a flyswatter covered with fly guts.

It could have been tempting to compare my childhood stories about punishment to my feeling that the leukemia was a form of retribution for my past indiscretions. However, I have never made that connection in my mind. Leukemia was simply a diagnosis.

CHAPTER 26

Indescribable Nausea

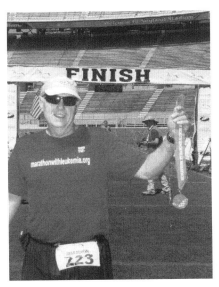

Covenant Health Marathon, Knoxville (2011)

God, grant me the strength to travel this distance,
the courage to push through the pain,
and the wisdom to know when to pick up the pace.
Anonymous

I returned from the Chevron Marathon in Houston on a Monday, and my first chemotherapy session was that Wednesday, February

2, 2011. I fear that will be one of those dates I will remember with clarity.

I showed up at the Mitchell Cancer Institute in Mobile at 7:30 a.m., signed in, and took a seat in the waiting room. Patients and family members occupied most of the seats. There were young and elderly men and women—white, black, and Asian. Cancer has no age, gender, or racial bias. For each of us, it attempts to deprive us of hope, steal our identity, and take away our passion.

The patients all had someone with them. Like at MD Anderson, I was alone.

I could not tell by looking at their faces if they were full of fear or of hope. I felt both. I feared that I would require a port for chemotherapy, and I feared how I would react to the impending chemical insult to my body. At the same time, I hoped that chemotherapy would help return me to something resembling my running ability before my leukemia diagnosis. It is more enjoyable running a marathon in the 3:30s than in the 5:30s.

The door to the infusion room opened. A nurse said, "Mr. Fields."

The wait and watch was over. The questions and worries that I had developed over the past three years were about to be addressed. The nurse led me to a chemotherapy station, and I took a seat in a comfortable recliner. Each recliner in the treatment room had an extendable footrest and was equipped with a computer for watching TV, searching the Internet, or reading e-mails. We exchanged the usual introductory comments while she went to work. Now came the moment I had been most anxious about: *Would the nurse find the veins around my wrist adequate for an intravenous line? Alternatively, would I need a port? Would I be able to continue running marathons in the next six months?*

As the nurse prepared to insert an IV line into my cephalic vein (a vein on the thumb side of the wrist), I prayed. Less than thirty seconds after she rubbed my wrist with alcohol and inserted a needle, she nonchalantly said, "This will work."

I blurted out, "Thank you, God."

My goal of running a marathon in all fifty states was still on. At least until I saw what chemotherapy was going to do to me.

Before attaching a chemical bag to my IV line, the nurse scanned my wrist ban. Next, she told me the names and amounts of the chemicals in the bag. I carried a note pad with the list of drugs and their amount, and I always compared this to what the nurse was reading. I did not want them infusing me with an improper chemical or too much of the correct chemical.

The infusion on Wednesday took almost eight hours. The nurse explained that if the infusion rate of rituximab was too fast, I might develop rigors, or die due to multifocal leukoencephalopathy (inflammation of the brain's white matter).

I inquired, "Do I need a mouth guard to prevent me from biting off my tongue?"

"No", she answered.

I tightly gripped the armrests anyway. I was expecting, at any moment, to look like Jack Nicholson in *One Flew over the Cuckoo's Nest*. I remembered the scene in which he went into rigors when given an electric shock treatment. Nothing happened, and I relaxed by grip.

Three hours later, the nurse hooked up the bag with the nasty concoction of fludarabine and cyclophosphamide. Over the next five hours, millions of cells were screaming as they exploded. No, I did not hear them, but I could sense the ghastly things those drugs were doing.

The Thursday and Friday infusions did not contain rituximab and only required five hours each day.

There were at least twenty patients in the treatment room at any one time. I watched various types of protocols for patients with different types of cancer. Some patients received a single injection in their abdomen, and others received a single infusion that took half a day. During my six months of chemotherapy, I did not see anyone getting the three-day treatment. I did not feel special.

The infusion room at the Mitchell Cancer Institute was not as primitive as the one in the book *Cancer Ward* by the Russian author, Aleksandr Solzhenitsyn. That story takes place on the oncology ward of a small hospital in Uzbekistan in 1955. It depicts how cancer transformed the daily existence of ten men. The horrors of Joseph Stalin's Soviet Union became insignificant when cancer entered their lives. The disease had become more important to them than any political system.

That book had created a lasting impression on me when I read it. Now I was living it. Leukemia had certainly transformed my life, and I was in a cancer ward receiving chemotherapy. Yet, unlike the ten men in Solzhenitsyn's book, my passion remained significant. Running had become even more important to me. It helped me feel normal while leukemia ravaged my physical being.

They referred to my protocol as emetogenic chemotherapy, a tasteful way of saying vomit-inducing chemotherapy. By Wednesday evening of each session, I was not able to keep anything down, not even water. The bad news was that I still had the Thursday and Friday infusions ahead of me. I spent the next four days becoming intimate with the toilet while throwing up.

Horrific does not begin to describe what I suffered Thursday through Sunday. When I was at the Mitchell Cancer Institute receiving chemotherapy, I wrapped myself in a blanket. At home, I had the heat cranked up and was under the covers suffering from chills. When I came home after a day of infusions, I remained in the fetal position. At times, the nausea was so bad that I believed I was on the verge of going into shock. I contemplated, *How long can I endure this?*

Over the weekend, I did not answer my phone and requested no visitors. I was too sick to move much less talk on a cell phone or entertain anyone at my apartment. Family and friends were not sure I had survived the weekend until I showed up for work or called them on Monday.

On Monday morning after that dreadful first weekend, I returned to the Mitchell Cancer Institute. The nurse collected a blood sample to see how the treatment was working. I did not need a blood test to answer that question. The first of the six planned chemotherapy sessions had nearly killed me. Consequently, I would have said that it was working very well.

They used the blood sample to see if the treatment had reduced my white blood cell count and that of the abnormal lymphocytes. Wow! Had it ever! My white blood cell count went from almost 200,000 per microliter to 50,000 per microliter after the first treatment.

They were also monitoring for tumor lysis syndrome (TLS), a metabolic complication that results from the rapid destruction of malignant cells. When cells die, they release their cellular contents into the bloodstream. (The adult male blood volume is approximately five liters. Therefore, I had almost one trillion dead cells circulating through my vascular system after the first round of chemotherapy.)

TLS can cause death by overwhelming the body's organs with dead cells. Therefore, I was told to drink three to four liters of fluid each day during and immediately after chemotherapy to help flush out the excess chemicals and waste. Of course, that did not happen. For four days, I could not keep anything down. Unfortunately, all that cellular debris was in my vascular and not my GI system. Otherwise, I could have thrown it up.

On Monday, I was fifteen pounds lighter than on the previous Wednesday, and I received fluid IVs. I would not recommend this diet.

Since chemotherapy destroys white blood cells, the nurse injected me with Neulasta to stimulate the bone marrow's production of neutrophils. These white blood cells help prevent bacterial infections. As the nurse injected the Neulasta, I inquired, "I'm in decent shape. How do elderly people who are not in shape survive the FCR protocol?"

"Some don't." "Others quit after the first treatment," she responded.

"Oh? I didn't realize that quitting was an option." Finally, someone laughed at my attempt at humor.

Importantly, the nurse removed that IV line. I now had sixteen days to look forward to feeling normal. Yet, as it would turn out, I would never return to normal and my goal post of normalcy would constantly be moving farther away.

Considering how sick I was during those four days, it amazed me how quickly my feeling sick dissipated. By Monday afternoon, I recovered sufficiently to lecture to the students and run after work. I now had to address an unanswered question: *Will I be able to run a marathon between chemotherapy sessions? Will I recover from the dehydration of chemotherapy and then a marathon in order to survive the next round of chemotherapy?*

There was no state in the month of February in which I had not run a marathon, so I scheduled two half marathons on consecutive weekends before my second chemotherapy session. On the first weekend, I ran the Rock 'n' Roll Mardi Gras Half Marathon in New Orleans (2/13/2011). The next weekend, I ran the Five Points of Life Half Marathon in Gainesville, Florida (2/20/2011). Other than the debilitating fatigue, everything seemed normal. I now felt confident that I could continue my goal in spite of chemotherapy.

Dr. Butler added something new for the second round of chemotherapy to combat the nausea. I applied a granisetron transdermal patch to my arm the day before the second round of chemotherapy. I suffered another four days with debilitating nausea.

Two weekends after my second treatment, Marian and I ran the Chesapeake Bay Running Club's Lower Potomac River Marathon in Piney Point, Maryland (March 13, 2011). My finishing time was 5:15. The trip was especially memorable. First, I did not think about chemotherapy for four whole days. Second, I proved to myself that I could complete a full marathon after having suffered through a chemotherapy treatment.

• • •

I received special treatment for my third chemotherapy session. I had my own private chemotherapy suite. (I later learned it was so that my vomiting would not disturb the other patients.) I again spent four days in the fetal position and felt I would not survive.

Two weekends after the third treatment, on April 3, 2011, Marian and I ran the Covenant Health Marathon in Knoxville, Tennessee. I lived up to the new nickname that The Team had given me, "Phil-Up-Chuck". My finishing time was 5:38.

After three sessions of chemotherapy, I became very weary. Chemotherapy had seriously challenged my will to continue. Showering was exhausting, preparing breakfast was exhausting, and standing for a lecture was exhausting. I was now operating on survival instincts: Survive the next round of chemotherapy and then survive the next marathon. Chemotherapy and running marathons were extracting an enormous physical toll from me.

One day while lacing my shoes for a run, I told myself, *If I cannot complete my run today, I will call it quits for now and rethink my timetable.* I then recalled something I had read, about the distinction between "to feel" and "to choose." I considered the following, *I feel like quitting. However, do I choose to quit? I have battled leukemia's attempt to rob me of my identity for over three years. Do I really want to stop now?* I convinced myself to continue the fight, and for another day, that was enough.

For my fourth chemotherapy session, Dr. Butler prescribed four additional antinausea drugs for the chemotherapy cocktail: Zofran, Reglan, Decadron, and diphenhydramine. I was now receiving eight antinausea drugs for the remaining three chemotherapy sessions: These drugs were only slightly more effective than eating M&M candy. There are no adjectives to describe how awful I felt. The less I moved, the less I seemed to hurt, but hurt I did. There were times that I would pinch myself to be sure I had not died and gone to hell.

• • •

After treatment five, Marian and I ran the Famous Idaho Potato Marathon in Boise, Idaho, on May 14, 2011. At this marathon, we parked at the finish, and volunteers bused us to the start. Arriving at the start, I realized that I had left the support for my torn gastrocnemius muscle in the car. There was no way I could run 26.2

miles without it. I boarded a bus that was going back to pick up more runners. Unknown to me, the bus was picking up runners for the half marathon. By the time I returned, the marathon runners were gone. I had to wait thirty minutes and start with the half marathoners.

This was not a chip-timed marathon, and my recorded finish time was 6:06. Surprisingly, I was not the last marathon runner to cross the finish line.

The day after the marathon, Marian and I rode the Thunder Mountain Train into the Idaho countryside. The tracks ran along the Payette River. A lush green valley was in the foreground, and snowcapped mountains were in the distance. We enjoyed a steak dinner in the dining car while the train went clickety-clack, clickety-clack down the track. For the moment, tranquility had returned.

• • •

From my private infusion room, I would occasionally hear a bell, so I inquired about it. The nurse informed me that when a patient completes the final chemotherapy session, the patient steps up and rings the bell. By Friday of my final session, I was too nauseous to participate in this tradition.

Two weeks later, on June 4, 2011, Marian and I celebrated the completion of my sixth and final chemotherapy session by running the Sunburst Marathon in South Bend, Indiana. Upon reaching the aid station at mile 20, the course marshal black-flagged (stopped) the marathon because of the heat. There were too many runners sent to hospitals because of heat stress. The marshal told us to stop running and wait for a bus that would transport us back to the start. All aid stations to the finish had shut down.

We waited thirty minutes for the bus to arrive, not to board the bus, but for a diversion. While the course marshal was pre-occupied with getting runners aboard the bus, Marian and I each grabbed a water bottle and snuck back onto the course. We had come too far not to finish. There were five other runners with the same idea.

As we entered the Notre Dame Stadium of the Fighting Irish, volunteers were dismantling the finish line. They gave us finisher medals so that we would have proof that we had run a marathon in Indiana. Thankfully, one of the volunteers gave us a ride back to the starting line and to our car. Our finishing time, counting the delay, was 6:30.

In bed that evening, I thanked God for granting me the strength to complete the marathons I had run during chemother-apy. Unknown to me, even more struggles lay ahead. I would again be humbled and asking God for help sooner than I anticipated.

CHAPTER 27
Humility versus Humiliation

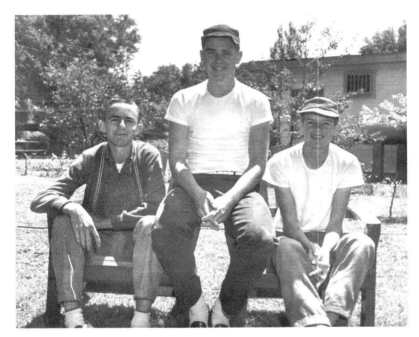

Left to Right: Warren Maddox, myself, James Smith (1962)

We learn humility through accepting humiliations cheerfully.
Mother Teresa[27]

Doctors report: "Runners are our worst patients. They think they can outrun their illness. They can't." I was a living poster child for that quote.

I had just recovered from the tear in my calf muscle, when I tore my left popliteus muscle (located behind the knee joint). It did not appear that I would ever run again without some sort of lower extremity wrap.

A friend said, "Leukemia is affecting your judgment. Who in their right mind runs when in pain or during chemotherapy?"

I could not adequately respond, especially since he could not possibly understand my passion for running. I could come up with only one logical response: "I cannot stop now. I am too close to the finish and cannot afford to let a little injury get in the way."

Actually, I was afraid to stop. I appeared to be breaking down physically, and was afraid I would not be able to start back again. James Van Praagh once said, "If you're on the path you're meant to be on, everything falls into place. If you are not on the right path, you will experience roadblocks all along the way, and this is the Universe telling you to stop, look, and ask if this is where you are supposed to be."[28] I did not think the universe was telling me anything, but maybe God was.

Fortunately, there was no marathon in July 2011 in a state that I had not run. I took a much-needed break to let my body heal from chemotherapy and to reflect on the path I was taking. I briefly pondered if God was telling me to stop. I reasoned that He was not, since my passion was not negatively affecting anyone else. Thus, I continued down the path toward my goal.

• • •

During my July break, I had a third bone marrow biopsy. Dr. Butler wanted to see if any abnormal lymphocytes remained. This would answer the questions, *Did chemotherapy work, and am I in temporary remission?*

Chemotherapy had caused a condensation of my hip bone marrow cavity. Thus, three trocar punches were required to extract sufficient bone marrow fluid for blood cell analysis. I mistakenly (or stupidly) refused the drugs again. Consequently, during the biopsy, there was facial flushing, contortions, sweating, and near fainting. Moreover, that was from the nurse watching me go through the ordeal.

I read the following from the literature: "Pain during a prior bone marrow biopsy creates anticipatory anxiety. Patients experiencing severe pain in the first biopsy are more prone to unbearable pain in the following one. A negative experience leads to fear and emotional distress for future biopsies." I laughed to myself as I continued to read. "Therefore, it is important not to traumatize the patient for future biopsies. A patient who experiences high anxiety before a biopsy tends to score higher levels of pain."

I thought, *Okay! The three biopsies have thoroughly traumatized me, and my anxiety level is through the roof. Next time I am requesting that they completely knock me out with anesthesia.*

After a week of restless anxiety, I was again sitting in Dr. Butler's office, waiting for the biopsy report. I thought back to the first time I had done this. Then, I did not know if I had leukemia or lymphoma. This time, I did not know if chemotherapy had worked. Sure, I knew the treatment knocked my blood counts below normal. Yet, I had no inkling if it rid my system of the abnormal lymphocytes.

As Dr. Butler entered the room, papers in his hand, I could immediately tell by his posture that the news was positive. I guess oncologists get excited when they can present their patients with good news. I liked Dr. Butler and was happy for him as he read the report, a smile on his face. "No abnormal lymphocytes present. You are in remission."

I wanted to shout "Halleluiah!" and dance around his office, although, I am too much of an introvert for that. Instead, I thought to myself, *Where is that bell? I want to ring that sucker.*

Going into chemotherapy, I was aware of the numbers. Only 45 percent of CLL patients who undergo FCR chemotherapy achieve remission. I am one of the lucky ones.

Whenever I think back to that six-month period of chemotherapy, I thank God for my being able to continue running marathons during treatment. I believe Sensei Ngo Dong would have been proud of me. I reached deep into my kiai, my inner strength, to accomplish that feat. Furthermore, like Mom had done so many years earlier, I looked a terrible adversity in the face and said, "Bullshit!" (Story in Chapter 32: Desire) I had not allowed leukemia to rob me of my identity and my passion or to impede my dream.

I could now look forward to four years of median progression-free survival (MPFS). MPFS is the average length of time my leukemia will remain in remission. Importantly, 78 percent of CLL patients were still alive five years after receiving FCR chemotherapy.

Unfortunately, the professor I had visited in Gainesville right before my own chemotherapy was not in the 78 percent group. His immune system never recovered after chemotherapy. After a little less than five years, he died from a bacterial infection in his lungs. I often recall my visit with him, overlooking the alligator-infested pond, and I say a prayer for him. He was a kindred spirit. We had both stepped off into the valley of the shadow of death praying for the best. I was the lucky one (**Chapter Related Memory: The Alligator.** The story is at the end of the chapter).

This underscores the fact that chronic lymphocytic leukemia is not curable and that it will return. Therefore, the wait and watch continued. Each month, a nurse stuck a needle in one of my arms to collect blood.

With chemotherapy in my rearview mirror, I had twenty-three states remaining on my list. Quitting at this time was not a skeleton in the closet from my past that I wanted to pull out and dance with again. Let me explain.

• • •

In 1961, 50 percent fewer high school students passed the physical exercise test than in the previous year. In 1962, President John F. Kennedy issued a challenge to the Marine Corps to walk fifty miles in full gear in twenty-four hours. The president hoped to jump-start a physical exercise program for people in the United States.

At the time of President Kennedy's challenge, I was in the ninth grade. Two high school friends (Warren Maddox and James Smith) and I decided to take the challenge. Our goal was to complete the fifty-mile hike in less than seventeen hours. We selected this time because it was a faster pace than President Kennedy's challenge. After all, we were young and fit, and we were not carrying full military gear.

We did not have the foggiest idea of what we were about to do or how to properly prepare. None of us had walked more than five miles at any one time. Regardless, we were enthusiastically ignorant. The route we measured was from Bushnell to Ridge Manor to Brooksville to Nobleton and back to Bushnell. We had hoped to do this without any fanfare. That way, if we failed, no one would know.

The three of us spent the night together so that we could get an early start. When we set out for Ridge Manor at 5 a.m. on Saturday morning, the local newspaper was there, taking our photos. Our parents had notified the news media. So much for no fanfare.

We each had an army canteen filled with water strapped to our belt. We also carried two sandwiches, which we stuffed into each of our back pockets. I do not recall what type of shoes my friends were wearing, but I was wearing my school loafers with thick white socks—not optimal walking gear.

We covered the first twelve miles to Ridge Manor ahead of a three mile-per-hour pace. We began to gloat: "This is not going to be so bad."

We refilled our canteens and struck out for Brooksville. There was not a cloud in the sky, the sun was heating things up, and we began to encounter hills. Still, we entered the city limits of Brooksville ahead of schedule but suffering from mild dehydration. We had walked the last five miles without water.

You would think that we would have picked a cooler time of the year to do this. Instead, we picked the middle of the summer. Consequently, we were going through our water every six miles. When we drove the course to get the mileage, we had failed to notice that there were no places between towns to get water.

We refilled our canteens in Brooksville and headed for Nobleton.

By now, the temperature was in the mid-90s, and the eleven miles to Nobleton was extremely hilly. The landscape only served to compound another oversight in our planning, which allows me to offer some advice: Do not attempt to hike fifty miles in blue jeans in the middle of the summer. By the time we walked into Nobleton, we were all suffering the worst chaffing from the jeans against our skin. Moreover, we still had twelve miles to walk.

We refilled our canteens in Nobleton and started the last leg of our journey to Bushnell. We were walking as if we each had a horse between our legs. Our bowlegged stance did little to relieve the chaffing pain. Two miles out of Nobleton, we could not take another step. Blood had stained the inner thigh areas of our jeans red. Stick a fork in us—we were done.

We sat under a tree for shade and discussed our options. We could suffer and complete the remaining ten miles, or we could admit defeat and hitchhike to Bushnell. While contemplating what to do, a Good Samaritan stopped and asked if we needed a ride. It is amazing how easy it was back then to accept defeat.

We got out of the Good Samaritan's car at the city limits of Bushnell and walked the remaining mile. (Unfortunately, he was going in the opposite direction or we would have ridden that mile as well.) During that last mile, we discussed what we would tell our parents. We agreed to tell them that we did not finish because the physical problems were too much to overcome. We would continue with, "Having learned from our mistakes, we will try again."

That was simple, straightforward, and the truth.

We approached our departure point sixteen hours after we had started. To our horror, our parents had planned a huge welcome home celebration. There was a large banner, a newspaper photographer, and all of our friends waiting for us. Again, two options confronted us: We could admit defeat, or we could lie.

The next day, our photo (the one at the beginning of this chapter) was in the *Sumter County Times* along with a story entitled, "Local Trio Gets into Hike Act." The article describes our successful completion of the fifty-mile walk in sixteen hours.

I did not get a restful sleep the next few nights. I later learned that my two friends had the same problem. We were all worrying about the same thing: Who would crack first and expose the lie? We were looking in the wrong direction. Remember, Mom was the county nurse and knew everyone in the county, and they all knew her. When the man who had given us the ride saw the article, he called Mom. It never occurred to us that he would be the one to spill the beans.

It has been so long that I do not recall all of the details. Nevertheless, I do remember that the newspaper published a retraction with our apology.

I learned an important lesson from that experience. Although it can be humbling, truth is the easiest way out of any situation. It may hurt initially, but in the end, it will spare a lot of anguish and humiliation.

Chapter Related Memory: The Alligator

I often recall my visit with Dr. Guillette overlooking the alligator-infested pond.

Michael and I once had a personal experience with an alligator. We were driving home from duck hunting on Lake Panasoffkee in Sumter County, Florida. A three-foot alligator was crossing the road. Michael stopped the car, grabbed the alligator by the tail, and swung it onto the back floorboard of Mom's car. Arriving back home, we went to the barn to make a place for Michael's latest pet.

That was when we heard the car engine start up. We ran to the front yard just in time to see Mom driving down the road toward town. She got about a quarter mile from the house when the car veered off into the ditch. Mom was out of the car almost before it had come to a complete stop. The alligator had managed to squeeze itself under the seat and between Mom's feet.

Michael always had a passion for animals. We were living in town, and, at the age of seven, Michael wanted a cow. Therefore, Mom and Dad bought ten acres of land and a cow. (This was the beginning of the ranch we called Jumper Creek Ranch.) The cow was a Jersey milk cow that Michael milked every morning before catching the school bus.

Mom insisted that Michael give the cow a name, so he named it Susie. From that day forward, Mom named every animal we ever had on our ranch. She named the cows, ducks, chickens, rabbits, and pigs. I believe the alligator's name was "Shit!" At least that was what we heard her call it as she leaped from her car.

CHAPTER 28

To Dream

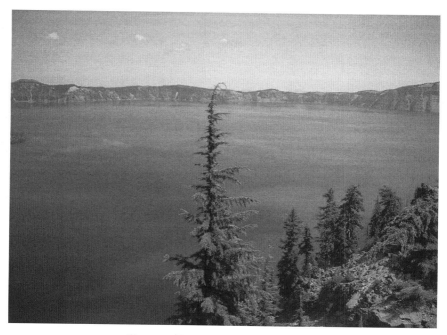

Crater Lake, Oregon (2011)

Never lose an opportunity of seeing anything that is beautiful,
for beauty is God's handwriting.

Ralph Waldo Emerson[29]

I consider myself blessed regarding chemotherapy. I never developed any bacterial or fungal infections in my lungs, or mouth sores. I did not have to use the special toothpaste or Miracle Mouthwash. I did not suffer from hematologic toxicity, tumor lysis syndrome (TLS), or hair loss. Except for four days of very bad nausea, things went fairly well. I say "fairly well" because there were some negative side effects that became evident over the next few years. The first side effect occurred during chemotherapy and for eight months after the last treatment. I had to get up and go to the bathroom every hour as though I had set an alarm. My sleep definitely suffered in those fourteen months. Although, I guess I can consider myself fortunate; I at least woke up in time to use the bathroom (**Chapter Related Memory: Peed 'n His Paa-yunts.** The story is at the end of the chapter).

• • •

My next marathon after the Sunburst Marathon in South Bend, Indiana (June 4, 2001), was The Crater Lake Marathon in Oregon on August 13, 2011. The course was, in part, on the road around the rim of the crater that had spectacular views of the lake. The first eighteen miles consisted of countless climbs up hills with inclines that lasted a mile or more. At a 7,000-plus elevation, this was my most challenging marathon.

On one extremely steep two-mile hill in the last four miles of the course, I stopped halfway up because I could not breathe. I simply stood there in the middle of the dirt road as if I were a cigar store wooden Indian. My body would not listen to my brain; I could not move. All of the runners who had passed me on the way up inquired of my status on their way back down. I was now the last runner. I eventually made it to the top and managed to pass one runner on the way down. My finishing time was 6:15.

Crater Lake is definitely the most beautiful spot that I have visited in our country. This spiritual place is undeniably one of

God's masterpieces. If you visit Crater Lake, book a room at Crater Lake Lodge. This is a magnificent lodge with a patio overlooking the lake.

Nearly 7,700 years ago, Mount Mazama erupted and then collapsed inward. This formed a crater that is five miles across. Later, the crater filled with water from rain and melting snow. At a depth of nearly 2,000 feet, this is the deepest lake in the United States. The brilliant aqua blue color is due to light rays penetrating into the depths of what is the purest water in the world. The blue wavelength reflects back and is what we see. The tops of the crater walls are more than 2,000 feet above the water level.

We enjoyed sitting on the patio in the quiet of the evening with a glass of wine. The night sky was perfectly clear since there were no city lights competing with the stars. The moon was full, and the Milky Way appeared as if it was close enough to touch. While looking onto the moonlit lake, I reflected on my blessed life and thanked God. If you do not leave Crater Lake a better person than when you arrived, something is terribly wrong—with you.

The Heart of America Marathon in Columbia, Missouri (September 5, 2011), is called the hardest nontrail marathon. The day was hot and the course was hilly, but I finished in 5:12.

Chemotherapy negated my shingles vaccination, and upon returning home, I ended up with shingles. Because of my zero immunity, oral acyclovir was not a treatment option. Instead, I spent a week in the hospital receiving the drug IV. The virus tracked along the branches of my trigeminal nerve, which provides sensory innervation to the face and orbit. The immunologist was concerned about the virus getting into my left eye and destroying my vision.

The virus destroyed the nerve endings on the left side of my face where the virus erupted, creating a sensation that ants were constantly biting me. They refer to this as postherpetic neuralgia. A prescription for Neurontin suppressed the sensation enough to allow me to sleep at night.

I had been on Neurontin for three months when I spoke to someone who had been on the drug for over five years. I happen to believe that being on medication for an extended period, unless needed for survival, cannot be good. Therefore, I began weaning myself from Neurontin by slowly cutting back on the daily dosage. Neurontin is very habit forming, and it took three months before I completely discontinued its use. The ants are still active, but I have learned to block them out mentally, at least enough to sleep at night.

I completed the Omaha Nebraska Marathon on September 25, 2011 in 5:08. This was a quick three-day weekend trip that I planned around my teaching schedule. Traveling alone, I did not do any sightseeing.

After chemotherapy, I was having trouble regulating my electrolytes (another effect related to the chemicals in the chemotherapy cocktail). Muscle cramps became a painfully common occurrence. At the Maine Marathon in Portland on October 2, 2011, my right calf muscles cramped at mile 11, and I could only hobble to the finish in 5:37.

The Des Plaines Trail Marathon in Illinois on October 10, 2011 was a nontechnical trail run in a forest. The trees were displaying their full fall colors and provided shade from the sun. At the beginning, the course went out one mile and then came back past the start/finish line. I did not complete a half mile before I developed cramps in my right calf muscles. I began hopping toward the side of the road and developed cramps in my left calf muscles. Since I am only a biped, I crumpled into a three-foot deep ditch with water.

Every runner inquired of my health as they ran past me to the one-mile turnaround, and again as they came back. I was still attempting to stand up without cramping. I felt like a land tortoise that was on its back, trying to turn over. I was finally able to stand up, and I started walking with intermittent jogging. Quitting was not an option. I could not afford any delays to my goal.

I finished with a time of 5:44 and won my age group. This time, I was not the only one in my 60-to-65 age group. I was 64.

The Route 66 Marathon in Tulsa, Oklahoma, on November 20, 2011 was another quick trip due to my teaching schedule. I finished the marathon in 5:11. It seemed like I would never run under five hours again.

The Honolulu Marathon in Hawaii on December 11, 2011 was the third time I ran in Hawaii, but it was my first time with leukemia. They still had the long aid stations with water, sports drinks, soft drinks, and sponges soaking in ice water. The sponges again reeked of BenGay and Tiger Balm by the time I reached them. My finishing time was 5:47.

Extreme fatigue continued to haunt me even after chemotherapy. The type of fatigue I experienced redefined "hitting the wall." This wall was nearly impenetrable. Everything in my body seemed to go into oxygen debt at the same time. I could not breathe and felt like I would collapse if I continued running. My body abruptly abandoned me—a total meltdown that came without warning. When this happened, I would force myself to run one-tenth to a quarter of a mile and then walk a short distance. This became my new normal.

Consequently, each marathon became a mystery. At the start line, I no longer had a finish time in mind. I simply asked God to help me get to the finish line. You may be asking why fatigue was still an issue after chemotherapy. The chemicals affected my bone marrow's ability to regenerate normal levels of white and red blood cells. A normal white blood cell count is 1,000 to 10,000 per microliter. Mine was 200 per microliter. A low normal red blood cell count is 4.5 million per microliter; mine was 3 million per microliter. I was getting into severe oxygen debt during marathons. (As of December 2018, my counts have not increased.)

I assumed or hoped that my running would improve after chemotherapy. Instead, I was struggling even more. There was no doubt that the chemicals in the FCR chemotherapy were a nasty assault on my body. The long-term negative side effects of overexposure to fludarabine and cyclophosphamide chemotherapy for CLL patients are destruction of bone marrow, heart problems, and death. When I considered that last option, I was thrilled to be able to continue my passion even if my times were slow.

The year 2011 ended with putting an additional thirteen states behind me. My average finishing time was 5:28, and only one marathon was under five hours: the First Light Marathon that I ran right before chemotherapy. It would be my last one under 5 hours.

It appeared that my road back to Boston had gotten longer. Nevertheless, I did not stop dreaming. In the words of James Van Praagh, "I'd rather look forward and dream, than look backward and regret."[30]

Chapter Related Memory: Peed 'n His Paa-yunts

I had to get up and go to the bathroom every hour as though I had set an alarm. Although I guess I can again consider myself fortunate; I at least woke up in time to go to the bathroom.

That jogged my memory about a humiliating event that could have been life changing, but was not. This event was so degrading that it is remarkable that I am not sitting in a wheelchair staring out a window into the abyss, overmedicated to control my behavior. I realize that is a bit of an exaggeration, but it was nevertheless a traumatic experience.

I was five years old and the youngest in my first-grade class. Five years old was excessively young to start first grade. At least, that was my opinion at the time. Looking back, I sometimes think, *Poor Mom. Each day she had to drag me screaming and hollering to the car in the mornings and drive me to school. Then she had to drag me from the car screaming and hollering and bring me into the classroom. It had to have been embarrassing for her, and it gives a completely new meaning to "unconditional love."*

To a five-year-old, the first-grade classroom looked massive. There were three long tables arranged in a capital 'I' formation. We sat in wooden chairs at these tables while the teacher walked around and checked our class work. The close proximity to cute girls in the class provided many opportunities for flirting. Of course, not yet having learned the proper technique for this, I was a nuisance and obnoxious.

One day, I raised my hand to get the teacher's attention. "What do you want, Mr. Fields?" she barked as she scowled at me. It was obvious that because of my previous behavior, I was not among her favorites. Feeling somewhat embarrassed for having to announce to the class my desire, I said, "I need to go to the bathroom."

"You were just at recess and should have gone then." She retorted.

Later, I raised my hand again.

"What is it this time, Mr. Fields?"

"I still need to use the bathroom," I said again, almost pleading since time was running out.

"I already answered you. Do not ask again, or I will send you to the principal's office."

I could feel my face turning beet-red with mortification.

The next single, solitary minute would haunt me for the remainder of my first grade year of school. I know that "single, solitary" is redundant, but it emphasizes what I am getting ready to convey. I wet my pants.

Imagine the indignity I suffered going to lunch with a huge wet spot on the front of my pants. The other kids were not sympathetic to my plight as they teased me the entire lunch period. Of course, the teacher made it even worse when I returned to class after lunch. In front of my classmates she said, "I see you wet your pants, Mr. Fields."

I had had enough of her! I countered, "Why do you call me Mr. Fields when my name is Phillip? It sounds like you are making fun of me."

"Don't you dare talk back to me!" she shrieked. "Get out of your chair and march right down to the principal's office."

As I walked to the principal's office, I contemplated my plight. *Oh great,* I thought. *Now even more people will see my wet pants and know what I have done.* To make matters worse, the principal moved a chair from his office to the hallway for me to sit in while waiting on Mom to come get me. I guess he did not want me sitting in his office since I smelled of urine.

Upon returning to school the next day, my classmates began taunting me, "Phillip peed'n his paa-yunts. Phillip peed'n his paa-yunts." By the end of the week, everyone in elementary school knew. Such an experience would alter the personality of most kids and warp their minds forever; I only sought retribution.

Payback was not long in coming. A few weeks later, the same thing happened: The teacher denied me a bathroom break. I had prepared for this moment and could not wait to put my plan into action. I slid my chair up close to the table, unzipped my pants, and peed on the floor. In the words of Colonel Hannibal in the movie *The A-Team*, "I love it when a plan comes together." However, unlike Colonel Hannibal, my plan was not perfect. I had failed to allow for trajectory and splash. Suddenly, the girl on the opposite side of the table from me jumped up, knocked her chair over, and started screaming, "Phillip peed on me! Phillip peed on me!"

I will never forget her stare, one of total disbelief at what had just happened to her. As I stared back at her, I thought, *You just had to say something. If only you had kept your mouth shut, this would likely have gone unnoticed until the janitor cleaned the room at the end of the day.*

Instead, I heard the teacher say, "Mr. Fields, you can just march yourself right down to the principal's office."

The school called Mom to come get me; the principal expelled me for three days. That was perfectly okay by me—I did not like school anyway.

CHAPTER 29
A New Hurdle

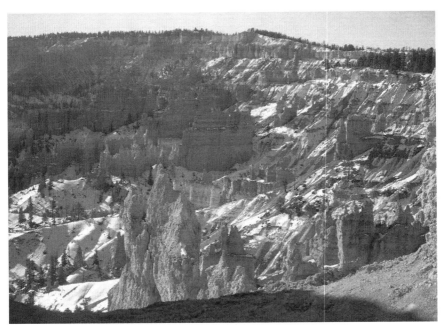

Bryce Canyon, Utah (2012)

*The parks are the nation's pleasure grounds
and the nation's restoring places.*

J. Horace McFarland[31]

With the beginning of 2012, I was close to the end of my goal. I
had thirteen states remaining in which I needed to run a marathon

in the next twelve months. I just hoped there would be no other medical issues to derail my plans. I hoped in vain, as it turned out.

My first stop for 2012 was the Running from an Angel Marathon in Boulder City, Nevada, just outside of Las Vegas on January 7, 2012. The race started at Lake Mead near the Hoover Dam. I finished in 5:37.

After the marathon, Marian and I drove to Zion National Park and hiked several trails into the mountains for views of the waterfalls and wildlife.

From Zion National Park, we drove two hours to Bryce Canyon where it was freezing cold, and everything was snow covered. We stopped at the visitor center on the way in, and the park ranger recommended that we go to the amphitheater over-look the next morning to see the sunrise. He also recommended that we purchase Pro-Yak tracks, which slipped over the bottom of our boots and would allow us to hike over ice and snow.

The next morning, the walkway to the end of the overlook was thick with ice, and walking without the Pro-Yak tracks would not have been possible. The wind was blowing twenty miles per hour, and the temperature was 14 degrees. Although I had bundled up, the freezing wind tore through my clothing as if I was wearing cheesecloth. If not for the ski mask, I believe my nose would have suffered frostbite. I was concerned that the moisture in my eyes would freeze.

With a full moon and the sky full of stars, this was another of those spiritual settings in which I reflected on my mortality and thanked God for a wonderful life.

As the moon was setting in the west, the sun slowly cleared the horizon in the east, casting its rays across the amphitheater below. A panoramic view of a massive gallery of snow-covered hoodoos (natural columns of rock in the western part of the United States that often are in fantastic forms) was the reward for our patience. I told myself, *Truly, there is a God.*

We drove back to the restaurant, thawed out with hot coffee, and had breakfast. We would need the fuel for our daylong hike into the bottom of the canyon. The temperature had warmed up to 16 degrees as we started our descent. It was so cold that the only sound was the crackling of snow and ice under our feet. Even the ever-croaking ravens were silent. We saw an amazing landscape of wind-carved rocks. Some had names: Queen Victoria and Thor's Hammer.

My second marathon in 2012 was the Birch Bay Marathon in Birch Bay, Washington, on February 19. Marian and I spent several days hiking different areas of the Olympic National Forest on our way to Birch Bay. Our first stop was Lake Quinault Lodge. The Quinault Rain Forest had moss- and lichen-covered trails along beautifully clear meandering streams. The only sounds in the forest were those of wonderful Mother Nature herself. There was an occasional fluttering of a bird's wings or the rustle of ferns as an unseen animal scurried about. We heard the quiet sound of a trickling stream as its water percolated over rocks and the thunderous sound of an occasional waterfall. Here we found the largest yellow cedar and Western hemlock in the United States and the world's largest Western red cedar, yellow cedar, mountain hemlock, Douglas fir, and Sitka spruce.

Our next stop was Kalaloch Lodge on the Pacific Ocean with hikes on Ruby Beach and Beach 4. Logs of fallen giants from the surrounding rain forest littered the water and beaches. While clambering around on the boulders at low tide, being careful to not fall into the water, we saw an amazing collection of sea anemones and starfish in the tide pools among the rocks.

From Kalaloch, we drove to Hoh Rain Forest with its moss-covered trees and a fern-carpeted floor. I had the feeling that if we lingered too long, moss would begin covering us as well. Except for the occasional sound of flowing water, the Hoh Rain Forest was dead silent. Moreover, the smell of dead fish permeated the air along the streams. Salmon had returned, spawned, laid their eggs, and were dying. Eagles and otters were having a grand feast.

My time at the Birch Bay Marathon was 5:05.

I developed pain in my sacral region during the marathon, but it did not seem to affect my training after returning home. I filed the incident away in the back of my mind.

Before the Napa Valley Marathon in California (March 14, 2012), Marian and I spent a couple of days touring wineries. We sampled wines at the Kunde Family Winery and at Deerfield Ranch Winery with its organic cave-stored wine. Lastly, we stopped at Castello di Amorosa, a medieval-inspired Tuscan castle with an extremely large yellow resident cat named Lancelot (twenty pounds of muscle). He was more than happy to climb up on my shoulders, where he stretched out and took a nap as we listened to the talk about the construction of the castle.

After sampling so much wine, I was almost pain-free for the marathon. I say *almost*. I could have used several more glasses of wine in order to stop the pain in my sacral area that again raised its ugly head. My finishing time was 5:27.

The day after the marathon, we took a short drive to Muir Woods. This is one of the country's oldest national parks, and it contains one of the last stands of old-growth redwood forest on earth. Some of the trees are 3,000 years old.

At the Ocean Drive Marathon, Cape May, New Jersey, on March 25, 2012, my sacral pain became so severe that I became nauseated and was throwing up. I still managed to finish the marathon in 5:38.

Our next marathon was the Salt Lake City Marathon in Utah (April 21, 2012). The day before the marathon, we walked to and around the Mormon Tabernacle property. The next morning at the start of the marathon, my sacral area was already throbbing. I made it to mile 10 but could not run any farther. Since there was not a time limit, I attempted to walk to the finish line. However, the pain was so intense that even walking was impossible. I caught a ride to the finish line aboard the sag-wagon. Fortunately, the hotel was just across the street from the finish area.

I had suffered my first DNF (did not finish), and I was angry and dispirited. Since 2009, I had never failed to finish a marathon, even during chemotherapy.

I spent the afternoon putting ice on the area and lying in bed, resting. The next morning we drove to Moab that is only a couple of hours from Salt Lake City. We spent the next several days hiking in Arches and Canyonlands National Park. There is nothing like a visit to a national park after a marathon to restore my health, mind, and soul. Luckily, the pain that had kept me from completing the marathon did not keep me from sightseeing. Probably because of the hydrocodone (600 mg) that I took after the marathon.

On the way to Moab is Dead Horse Point State Park. The canyon rim towers 2,000 feet above the confluence of the Colorado and Green rivers. The park got its name from a legend, a rather bleak one at that. Cowboys rounded up and corralled wild mustangs into a fenced area. They selected the best mustangs for their personal use, and they left the rest corralled. Those left behind died of thirst within view of the Colorado River. I certainly hope this was just a legend.

We spent the next two days hiking in Arches National Park where trails led to some of the more spectacular 2,000-plus sandstone arches. A favorite hike was to Delicate Arch. If you are brave enough to hike out onto the slope, you can look through the arch at the salt canyon below. Where did the salt come from? This area is part of the Colorado Plateau that includes Utah, Arizona, New Mexico, and Colorado. The sea covered the plateau 300 million years ago and left a huge salt deposit.

The primitive trail in Devil's Garden was our most arduous hike. You reach a point on the trail where you have a choice. If you feel some passageways are only fit for animals with feathered wings, stop. Yet, if you have the feet of a mountain goat, finish hiking the primitive trail to get even more views of outstanding arches.

The Green and Colorado rivers separate Canyonlands National Park into three land districts: Island in the Sky, The Needles, and The Maze. Island in the Sky and The Needles are the easiest to access and are the ones Marian and I hiked. Several trails led to ruins and pictographs of Ancient Pueblo people who once inhabited the area. Like the Arches, the Permian Sea covered the area at one time.

(On a related note: When you go hiking in the parks, I advise that you stay on the marked trails. The ground is alive with cyanobacteria. This blue-green alga creates black carpets across the landscape that provide a foothold for plant growth. These carpets take centuries to develop, and one footstep can destroy them in a second.)

When I returned to Mobile, it was time for my monthly blood sampling. I discussed the sacral pain with Dr. Butler, and he ordered an MRI. I had a fractured sacrum. Without any known trauma to create such a fracture, the orthopedic oncologist was concerned that the fracture was due to a metastasis and he ordered a CT scan. Fortunately, there were no bone masses. The orthopedic oncologist said it would take four to six months for my sacrum to heal. He gave me a prescription for crutches in order to take weight off the fracture.

There would be no running during the healing process. This time I followed the doctor's advice. I canceled three plane flights to our May and June marathons. Now, my marathon schedule was in shambles. I was running out of months in which to complete the states by the end of the year. I made some mental calculations: *If I go three months without running that will take me to the end of July. That will be just in time to run the Juneau Alaska Marathon.* I had long ago registered for that marathon and I was not about to cancel that trip.

I studied the calendar. Because of my teaching schedule, I could not travel in August or November. Consequently, after the marathon in Juneau, Alaska, I would need to run seven marathons in September, October, and December in order to finish the states by the end of the year. This was a tall order.

I contemplated the uncertainties: *Will my sacrum heal enough in three months so that I will be able to run in Alaska? After all, the doctor said four to six months. Will the remaining states line up properly for September, October, and December? How well will my sacrum tolerate my running seven marathons in three months? Will I be physically able to do this? After all, running just one marathon each month has become stressful to my body.*

More than one friend inquired, "Why not back off and take proper time to heal? Spread the remaining states out over next year." From the looks in their eyes, I believed they were considering sending people in white uniforms to carry me off in a straightjacket. There was no way I could provide a logical answer that they would appreciate. Simply put, I am a goal-oriented person, and from the very beginning, my goal was to complete marathons in all fifty states by the end of December 2012. There would be no compromising.

At this point, my thoughts were as follows: *This is the fifth year since my diagnosis. What if the oncologist at MD Anderson was correct and I only have five to seven years left. What if all the injuries I have suffered since chemotherapy are the beginning of a downward spiral? I cannot take that chance and procrastinate with the remaining states.*

If nothing else, remaining active was preferable to sitting home in a comfortable chair watching bad movies and waiting for the sand to empty from my hourglass.

CHAPTER 30
The End is in Sight

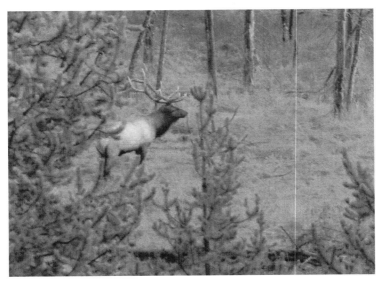

Bull Elk, Yellowstone National Park (2012)

When defeat comes,
accept it as a signal that your plans are not sound,
rebuild those plans,
and set sail once more toward your coveted goal.

Napoleon Hill[32]

The Frank Maier Marathon in Juneau, Alaska, on July 28, 2012 was my first run after twelve weeks of healing my fractured sacrum.

Fortunately, there was only a slight discomfort in my sacrum during the marathon. I finished in 5:47.

The day after the marathon, Marian and I drove to the Mendenhall Glacier, where we hiked trails through lush foliage and along salmon-filled streams. This was salmon-spawning season, and the streams were alive with the salmon's playful courtships.

The park ranger gave us a warning: "Do not hike with an open bottle or bag of food because of bears in the area. Stores sell bells that you can tie to your shoes to prevent walking upon an unsuspecting bear. The bear will generally leave the area when it hears the noise. Stores also sell garlic spray for your clothes. Bears do not like the smell of garlic." The park ranger also informed us: "You can tell what a bear has been eating by looking at the bear's scat. It may contain various types of wild berries, or it may contain bells and smell like garlic." Although we came across fresh bear scat, I did not stop to smell it and I did not see any bells.

Eagles were everywhere. These magnificent birds were flocking to the area for their yearly salmon feast. Following their cue, we enjoyed eating some ourselves (salmon, not eagles). We sampled Sockeye, Coy, and my favorite, King. The halibut was even better than the salmon.

Gustavus was only a short plane ride from Juneau. For a reasonable price, we reserved lodging at Glacier Bay Lodge and a day cruise up Glacier Bay. At the lodge, there was a porcupine in a cottonwood tree eating leaves. Who would have thought a porcupine climbed trees? You do not want those needles raining down on you. Near the lodge, there were several hiking trails through forests, along meandering streams and past hyacinth-covered water sheds. While hiking through this silent prehistoric-looking forest in a drizzling rain, I expected to see a Tyrannosaurus Rex at any moment.

The Glacier Bay cruise ship was small enough to get close to the shoreline. This put us within camera range of a black bear, a couple of brown bears with their cubs, a family of black wolves basking in the sun on a beach, and mountain goats on the side of cliffs. During the cruise, we also spotted humpback whales, sea otters, and orca. The boat took us right up to Johns Hopkins, Lamplugh, and Margerie Glaciers. Waves produced by large chunks of ice breaking off and falling into the water (calving) created a graceful rocking of our boat.

The glaciers are an exquisite turquoise blue because the ice is so dense that it absorbs all colors of the spectrum except blue. This color reflects back and is what we see, similar to Crater Lake.

I now had seven states left in which to run marathons but only three available months. In order to finish by December 2012, I would have to run a marathon on three consecutive weekends in September and again in October. There was no turning back. The finish line was just around the corner. I did not have room in my schedule for any more injuries or DNFs.

On September 8, 2012, I traveled alone to a little-known town in Utah. Huntington is a tiny town with a main street, three streetlights, one restaurant, and one motel. It is the home of the Little Grand Canyon Marathon.

The Little Grand Canyon was not as breathtaking as the Grand Canyon, but it was impressive just the same. While driving along the canyon rim, I stopped at numerous overlooks, where I had panoramic views. I did not realize it at the time, but I was looking down onto where I would be running the next day.

This was a point-to-point marathon, in which the starting and finishing lines are 26.2 miles apart. The first 18 miles went through open country. The ground and sky blended in the distance. With a scarcity of trees and a lack of shade, the sun was merciless. Around mile 18, the road turned into an area with huge rock formations on either side. This was San Rafael Swell, or Buck Horn Wash, and is what I had been looking down on from the canyon rim the day before.

The towering red rocks are a geological timetable. I was now running through the Jurassic, Triassic, and Cretaceous Eras. This was a dream come true for a former youngster who had aspired to be an archeologist. At one point, we ran by fossilized dinosaur footprints on the side of the road.

I was way behind other runners, and I was running alone through this primitive area. Back when I was a young archeologist wannabe, I often wondered if dinosaurs still inhabited isolated areas of our earth, impossible though that may be. Now I questioned, *Will I encounter a Velociraptor as I round one of these many blind curves on this canyon road?* Fortunately, there were no such sightings.

My fantasizing only briefly distracted me from the agonizing heat. The temperature in the floor of the canyon was over 90 degrees. Heat was reflecting off the canyon wall like that off an AstroTurf football field. The only shade I found was that formed by tumbleweeds. The debilitating effects of cancer-related fatigue, my low red blood count, the heat, and the high elevation (5,000 feet) made it difficult for me to put one foot in front of the other and move forward. Yet, failure at this point in my journey was not acceptable. I prayed and pushed on.

In the last five miles, the course went by a large panel of Native American pictographs. They were on the face of one of the towering rocks beside the road. I tried to imagine what the artists were thinking when they made those drawings. *What was it like living back then in such a hostile environment?*

I began to view myself running a marathon 10,000 years in the future. In my mind, I ran through the remains of a prehistoric city and came across some pictographs. These were spray-paint drawings on the sides of ruined buildings, a railroad car, and a bridge piling. Unable to interpret their meaning, I wondered, *What was it like living back then in such a hostile environment?*

This latest diversion worked. I had again managed to defeat the circumstances of the moment and complete another marathon. My finishing time was 6:21, and I was not last. As much as I suffer during a marathon, I cannot imagine what those behind me must feel.

This was the first of three consecutive marathons that would each take me over six hours to complete: This one was because of the heat and elevation. The next one would be because I converted the marathon into an ultramarathon. The third was because it was as fast as I could go.

I traveled alone to the Kroll's Marathon in Bismarck, North Dakota (September 15, 2012), and volunteered to help at the packet pickup. It was a great way to give something back to those who worked so hard to satisfy my addiction.

Knoll's would be my first ultramarathon, although I would not be able to count it as an ultramarathon. Let me explain. Any distance greater than 26.2 miles is an ultramarathon. There is one important requirement, though: You have to plan the distance at the beginning of your run. I certainly did not intend to run more than my allotted 26.2 miles.

So how did I manage to convert this marathon into an ultra-marathon? The course had a short two-mile loop at the start, followed by a long out-and-back loop. Then you reran everything. On the return from the longer loop, I correctly ran around the outside of the initial short loop. However, at mile 13, I was supposed to turn left toward the finish line and repeat the short two-mile loop. Instead of turning left and repeating the short loop, I continued straight ahead, thinking I had done the short loop by running the outside area.

I was not aware of my error until mile 16, when I noticed that the mileage on my Garmin watch did not match the mile marker. I backtracked 1.5 miles, ran the short loop that I had missed, and ended up running 29.2 miles. My time was 6:19.

I was not the only ignoramus that day. The female winner (or at least the woman they thought had won) made the same mistake but never realized that she had done so. The difference was she was trying to win the race and I was just trying to finish.

The Jackson Hole Marathon (September 23, 2012) starts in Jackson, Wyoming. Jackson is a town in Jackson Hole (a valley carved out by a glacier). With an elevation of over 6,000 feet, I struggled to a 6:19 finish.

The next day, Marian and I went sightseeing in the Grand Teton National Park just outside Jackson. We photographed a family of moose, a frisky beaver in a pond, and a bull elk on a hill. We completed a four-hour hike to Hidden Fall and Inspiration Point. The trail went along Jenny Lake, where the fall foliage was a lavish expression of artistic creation. Simply put, the leaves were beautiful.

After another evening of eats and relaxation in Jackson, we drove to Yellowstone National Park. Old Faithful Lodge is centrally located in the park, and staying there saves a lot of driving time. We spent four days hiking at Old Faithful, Norris Geyser Basin, the Grand Canyon of the Yellowstone, and Mammoth Hot Springs near the northern entrance to the park. Yellowstone is teeming with buffalo, elk, wolves, and moose. September was elk rutting season and the trumpeting sounds from bull elks filled the air with their love melody.

Words cannot accurately describe Yellowstone National Park. There are hiking trails past spewing, bubbling, gurgling, and hissing geysers, not to mention fumaroles, mud pits, and colorful hot springs. While being enthralled by all this energy, I remembered I was standing on top of a caldera of molten lava that is so massive that should it erupt, it would most likely destroy most of North America. There is a movie, *2012,* which has great cinematography and depicts the (fictitious) eruption of the Yellowstone Caldera.

Hiking and sightseeing in our national parks has caused me to pause and marvel at God's marvelous creations. Without leukemia, these trips would never have happened. What a blessing!

I now had two weeks to prepare myself mentally for three more consecutive weekends of running marathons.

I traveled alone to the Amica Marathon in Newport, Rhode Island (October 14, 2012) and I again volunteered to help at the packet pickup. The marathon course went by the grand, gorgeous Newport mansions: the Breakers, Marble House, Rose Cliff, and The Elms. I finished the marathon in 5:30.

The next weekend was The Des Moines Iowa Marathon (October 21, 2012), where I again volunteered at the packet pickup. For most of this race, I ran behind three of the most unusual runners. One wore a backpack, which in itself is not strange, but the contents were. Around mile 5, one of the runners said, "I'm thirsty and ready for one." He reached into the backpack, pulled out a can of beer, popped the cap, and began drinking while running. Later, another runner said, "I'm ready for a smoke." She reached into that same backpack and pulled out a pack of cigarettes. She lit one up and began smoking while running.

Those three runners smoked cigarettes and drank beer the whole way, and they still finished in front of me (**Chapter Related Memory: Grape Vines.** The story is at the end of the chapter).

My finishing time for the Amica Marathon was 5:30.

The weekend after the Des Moines Iowa marathon I traveled alone to The Cape Cod Marathon in Falmouth, Massachusetts (October 28, 2012). The day before the marathon, I went sightseeing in the downtown area of Falmouth. Restaurants, shops, and light fixtures with hanging flower baskets lined both sides of the streets. Scarecrows also dotted the sidewalks. It was close to Halloween, and shop owners were dressed for the season. They were handing out candy to the young goblin-clad trick-or-treaters. A 50-State Club member that I met at the Little Grand Canyon Marathon told me to visit the Quarterdeck restaurant when I was in Falmouth. I did so and enjoyed an excellent cup of clam chowder and a lobster roll.

I finished the marathon in 5:30.

I had a full teaching schedule in November, and the month-long break from running a marathon was welcome after six marathons in eight weeks.

Connecticut was my last state. I had selected a little-known marathon in Roxbury, the Roxbury Marathon (December 8, 2012). There was not a lot to choose from because of the narrow window in my teaching schedule and the upcoming Christmas holiday.

It was hard to contain my excitement during the week leading up to the Roxbury Marathon. Yet, I remained cautious. I did not want to hear God's laughter. Not now, at least.

Chapter Related Memory: Grape Vines

Those three runners smoked cigarettes and drank beer the whole way, and they still finished in front of me.

I remember the first time I tried smoking. None other than Jackie Huggins initiated me. The tree where I built my treehouse had grape vines growing up into the limbs. The technique, as described by Jackie, was this: "Use the dead and dried grape vines, which are hollow. Next, light one end and puff away on the other end."

I was only ten years old, but I felt like I was twenty. That is, until I let the vine burn down too far, sucked fire into my mouth, and burned my tongue.

CHAPTER 31
Unfinished Business

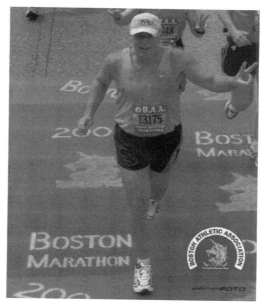

Boston Marathon (2004)

One thing robs me of my peace of mind:
A DNF (Did Not Finish) at the Boston Marathon.

Phillip Fields

On race day at the Roxbury Marathon (December 8, 2012), there was a bit of a chill in the air. The first six miles were over rolling hills and a dirt road, Judd's Bridge Road. The turnaround was at

Judd's Bridge, which led to Judd's Bridge Farm, a picturesque farm with a large red barn, silo, and farm equipment parked in the barnyard. I struggled going up the front side of the steep inclines those first six miles. Of course, I had the opportunity to experience the backside of them during the return. The next portion of the race consisted of five loops of more hills. Therefore, I experienced each hill five times.

The smell of fresh cow manure was in the air. I thought about Fred Greenwood, our visits at the Society for the Study of Reproduction meetings, and my research sabbatical at the University of Hawaii in Honolulu (1994).

At the finish line, there was no announcement or fanfare for my accomplishment of completing a marathon in all fifty states. I did not wear a sign that indicated my achievement. Other than Marian and me, no one knew. That was the way I preferred the ending.

The last marathon in my fifty-state journey was significant in three ways. First, it was the last state. Second, it took me the longest time to complete, 6:29. Third, this was the only marathon that I finished last. Let me explain the third significance.

Marian was running with a hamstring injury, and I ran with her to keep her company. We were definitely going to be the last two finishers. During the run, I contemplated, *Should I be chivalrous and let Marian cross the finish line ahead of me? I have run marathons with leukemia, torn muscles, a fractured sacrum, with the flu, and during chemotherapy. I have suffered through a lot of pain and a lot of puking. This has been an amazing four-year journey, a testament to what the body and the mind can overcome when called upon to do so. Yet, in spite of everything, I have never finished last. This is the last marathon of my goal. Do I want to give up this record?*

As I approached the finish line in the final loop, it was decision time. My final thought was, *I could not have completed this goal without Marian there to help lift me up through so many difficult times.* Therefore, I let Marian cross the finish line ahead of me. This was the first marathon in which I was the last runner to complete the marathon—but wait, they mixed up the pull tags and listed Marian as the last runner. The results listed me as next to last. How funny is that?

* * *

When I returned to Mobile, there was no ticker tape parade. There was no congratulatory sign or reporter as there had been in 1962 for that fifty-mile walk. This was only because Mom was not around to arrange the celebration. She would definitely have used that opportunity to brag about her son. I used to hate when she did that. Now, I miss her not being around to do so.

If she were here, I would give her a big hug and a big thank you for my ability to complete this goal. Her memory and inspiration were always present during this journey. Looking back at my childhood, I believe she may have inspired me to run. When I was in elementary school, I remember her running laps around one of our cow pastures. Had she lived in Mobile, Alabama or Gainesville, Florida she would probably have run races.

Back at work the day after the Roxbury Marathon, it finally clicked: I had actually run a marathon in every state and Washington, DC. My thoughts traveled back to 2008 when the oncologist at MD Anderson told me not to run because of the horrible things that might happen. Yet, having repeated Florida, I ran fifty-two marathons in forty-seven months. Sure, I suffered numerous injuries along the way, but I did not endure any of the insults described by the oncologist—except for the nausea and fatigue.

So where is the euphoria? Why am I feeling such melancholy? I asked myself.

The answer was unfinished business. When I began my goal of running a marathon in every state, I secretly hoped that the Boston Marathon would be among the fifty. After training for and running all those marathons, I figured I would qualify again for Boston. When I set that goal, I never fully appreciated how difficult it would be with leukemia.

Returning to Boston would have gotten the monkey off my back, so to speak. What monkey you ask? I told the story of qualifying for the 2004 Boston Marathon in Chapter 13, "Counting Marathons." You may have realized that there was no discussion about that trip. That is because I was a DNF. That failure has haunted me ever since.

Some of you may be saying, "Hey, it is only a race. Forget about it and move on." There were times I wish I could have done so. Since I first learned about the Boston Marathon on a bus ride back in 1985, it has been the paramount marathon for me. My desire to qualify and complete this race was nothing less than that of the medieval knights' quest for the Holy Grail in the Arthurian legends.

I will never forget the wonderful memories of the 100th Boston Marathon. However, that DNF in 2004 created an itch that I could not scratch. More than once, Dad would say, "A job worth beginning is a job worth finishing." Boston was unfinished business.

So, what happened at the 2004 Boston Marathon?

Don "The Stallion," Mike "Mad Dog," and I traveled to Boston and checked into a hotel within walking distance of the Boston Common. On the morning of the marathon, we rode one of the hundreds of school buses to Hopkinton. I felt as much excitement as I had in 1996. After all, this was the Boston Marathon.

The marathon still had a noon start. In fact, almost everything was as I remembered it in 1996. There was one big difference: The temperature was a record high for the race start, a hot 85 degrees. I viewed this difference as a positive. In 1996, the temperature had been in the 30s, it had been raining, and the Wellesley women had been bundled for the weather. In 2004, I remember thinking, *When I get to the scream tunnel, those ladies will be scantily clad.*

When I reached the scream tunnel, I was not disappointed. The amorous Wellesley women were dressed for the heat. As I had done in 1996, I moved to the right side of the road. Again, the women fondled me as if they were shopping for a ripe cantaloupe. Like in 1996, I departed that area with an adrenaline rush.

Early on, it was obvious that the heat was going to influence the race. Runners were down everywhere along the course. Some runners were on the side of the road with leg cramps, others were throwing up on the course, and more were in Red Cross tents.

When I crossed the timing mat at mile 13.1, photographers were taking photos from a platform above the mat. I raised my left arm with my fingers in the victory sign (Photo at the beginning of the chapter). The excitement of the Boston Marathon had me pumped and the heat had gone unnoticed. I felt great, misleadingly so.

That year, there were no drums at the top of Heartbreak Hill. However, the crowd was there to taunt anyone who stopped and walked up. When I reached the top around mile 21, I was ahead of schedule to qualify for the 2005 Boston Marathon. I had time for a necessary pee stop at the port-o-lets at the top of Heartbreak Hill. When I reached them, they were all in use. I waited since I had time to spare.

That was the last thing I remembered until I came to on the grass next to a Red Cross tent. Red Cross workers had packed ice bags beside me. Apparently, I had passed out in front of the port-o-let. It is a good thing runners occupied all the port-o-lets. I could have entered, locked myself in, and probably not been found until workers emptied it the next day.

I moved to get myself off the ground in order to reenter the marathon. My right calf muscles cramped. I lay back down until the cramps subsided. I tried again, and my muscles in both calves cramped. Then my pectoralis muscles cramped as I tried to pull myself up using an army cot next to me. I overturned the cot with its occupant. Every time I tried to move from the ground, something cramped. I needed someone to get behind me and lift me straight up like a board so I did not have to bend anything.

I asked the people at the Red Cross tent to help me up, but they would not assist me. They said I needed to stay put until an ambulance arrived. I responded: "Ambulance? That is nonsense. It is only cramps," I pleaded, but they ignored me.

Eventually, I saw soldiers approaching. I was not hallucinating. A group of soldiers was marching in formation the entire course. I called out to them. I felt excited, thinking, *They will be able to get me up, and I will finish the marathon with them.* As they began to lift me off the ground, the Red Cross workers came over and stopped them.

With the passing of the soldiers, the end of the race had to be near. I began to panic. The finish line was only five miles away. However, every time I tried to move to get up, something would cramp.

When the emergency medical technicians (EMTs) arrived, my chance of getting off the ground and finishing the most prestigious marathon had ended. The EMT personnel rolled me onto a stretcher and carted me off to a hospital somewhere in Boston. There were so many runners at the hospital that they had us on gurneys in the hallways. Everyone had IVs going.

(Don) "The Stallion," (Mike) "Mad Dog," and I were supposed to get together that evening for dinner with other runners from Mobile. I had written Don's cell phone number and the name of our hotel on the back of my bib with a dry erase pen. When I arrived at the hospital, the writing was nothing more than an ink spot. I panicked. Fortunately, when I failed to show up at the hotel, Don began calling all the hospitals in Boston. He claimed he first called the morgues—funny guy. It was amazing that he located me.

After four bags of IV fluids, the doctor released me. I caught a cab back to the hotel. The door attendant paid the cabbie, and I later reimbursed the hotel attendant with a tip.

I did not want the above memory to be my last one of the Boston Marathon. Hence, the unfinished business that marred my fifty-state accomplishment.

CHAPTER 32

Desire

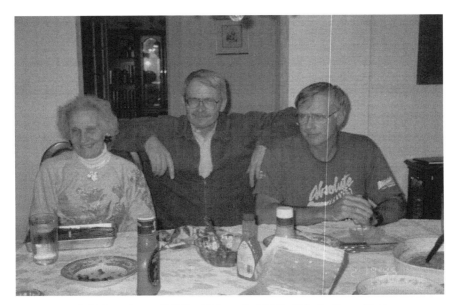

Mom, Michael, and Me (Mom's 77th Birthday, February 20, 1993)

Hope is not a dream,
but a way of making dreams become a reality.

L. J. Suenens[33]

After forty-seven months, torn muscles, chemotherapy, and a fractured sacrum, I had completed a marathon in all fifty states and

Washington, DC. Throughout the journey, I thought about Mom and mentally thanked her for setting an example of toughness. I contemplated, *What I endured these past forty-seven months was only a microcosm of what she overcame.*

I will explain. In March 1999, Mom was putting out cattle feed and hay at the age of eighty-three when she suffered a stroke. The infarct was in the left middle cerebral artery, which supplies an area of the brain that controls speech and motor nerves to the right side of the body, her dominant side.

When the neurologist came to her bedside after all of the clinical tests that he had requested had been performed, he callously told her that she would spend the rest of her life confined to a bed. I was stunned into silence, and I thought, *How can you be so insensitive and shatter all of my mother's hope?*

I believe Mom felt the same way because she managed to tell him, "Bullshit!" She was a true cattle woman. It would be four months before she was able to speak again.

After a brief period at UF Health Shands Hospital, the doctors moved Mom to Shands Rehabilitation Center. Many of the patients at the rehabilitation center had no visitors. As I sat and watched these patients, I asked myself, *Do they have family or friends? Does their physical condition make it too uncomfortable for family or friends to visit? Did their neurologist also tell them that their condition would confine them to a bed for the rest of their lives? If so, they probably do not feel like they have anything to live for. Without hope, how can they be optimistic and aspire to something better? How can they dream of recovering?*

As depressing as MD Anderson was, it never matched the dispiriting atmosphere of that rehabilitation center.

My brother lived in Gainesville and visited Mom every day. I drove down once each month for a long weekend visit around my teaching schedule. It was difficult to watch Mom, who had been so active, confined to a bed. Although I am sure that Mom's anxiety was more than ours was. As it turned out, her faith was stronger also. She had hope and a desire: seeing her dog and her cows again.

I quickly discerned the routine of the physical therapists at the rehabilitation facility. They would give their patients a series of exercises to do on their own. Later, the therapists would return to help the patients with a more extensive workout. Many patients would not complete or even begin the initial exercises. When the therapist returned, these same patients would say, "I don't feel like doing anything today." Sadly, it was not long before the therapists stopped putting forth much effort to help these patients. After all, if you are not willing to help yourself, no amount of effort from others can help you.

Not so with Mom. She quickly completed the initial exercises. If her physical therapist did not return in a timely fashion, she would do them again. After seeing Mom's enthusiasm, the therapist began giving her more exercises to do on her own. When the therapist returned, he would spend more time with Mom on tasks that were even more difficult.

Mom enjoyed having me present during physical therapy. She thrived on showing off the small gains that she was making in her recovery. I mean *small* gains. At that time, she could not use her right side, could not speak, and had trouble swallowing. Although, the fire in her eyes and that now-crooked smile on her face never faded. One day, I told Mom that her smile reminded me of Uncle Lester. He had served in World War I, and a mortar shell had exploded near him. He, too, had a crooked smile

(Chapter Related Memory: Strawberry Short Cake. The story is at the end of the chapter).

Without a family that cares, most stroke patients will spend their remaining days in an assisted-living facility. There is no way that a patient who has had a severe stroke will recover with only physical therapy offered through insurance. Even with a family's help, it is not certain the patient will ever be able to care for themselves.

After Mom had spent a month at the rehabilitation center, Michael took her into his home. Taking care of Mom was a 24/7 job. My brother's wife, Margaret, accepted this change in their family routine as if Mom was her own mother. A caregiver spent the day with Mom while Michael and Margaret were at work. She helped Mom with physical therapy, walking exercises, and she prepared meals for the whole family.

After Mom had spent five months at Mike's, we changed the routine. Leslie and I lived in a two-story house in Montrose, Alabama. The bedrooms and two baths were downstairs, and the living area and kitchen were upstairs. This setup made it impossible for Mom to stay with us. Instead, we moved her to an assisted-living facility in Fairhope, Alabama, about ten miles from our home.

Mom went to physical therapy three days each week. She received physical therapy, speech therapy, and swallowing therapy. Regardless of how hard the therapists pushed Mom, she always wanted more. As she regained some of her ability to speak, she was able to share with us her goal that had made her so determined and strong: to be home with her dog and cows by Christmas. This was an ambitious goal. Christmas was less than one year from when the neurologist told Mom that she would remain bedridden for the rest of her days.

If Mom was going to achieve her goal, I needed to accelerate the rehabilitation process. Every evening after work and each day on the weekends, I would "descend like a vulture" (as Mom would describe it) on Mom with my workout bag of goodies. My bag contained dumbbells and ankle weights.

Our daily routine was for her to walk as far as she could, using a three-legged cane, to the game room where we exercised. I would pull a wheelchair behind me for when she could walk no further. The game room was thirty yards from her room. We were both excited the first day that she walked all the way. Before she left Fairhope, she was walking 100 yards with the cane.

In addition to her right side, which had been affected by the stroke, I had her exercise her left upper and lower extremities—the good side—the left side would be doing most of the work when she returned home.

Before Mom left Fairhope, she was able to lift her right leg (the affected side) with an ankle weight attached. She could also extend all of her fingers and wrist on her right side, although she never was able to do much with her right upper extremity.

I wish I could have talked her into staying one more month to work on writing with her left hand. However, her goal was to be home by Christmas, and she had no intention in deviating from that aspiration. I guess I learned from her about setting and not departing from a goal.

Mom's time in Fairhope was not all work. On several weekends, I took her to our home on Mobile Bay. We entered the ground floor where the bedrooms were located. She seated herself on a large pillow and blanket at the foot of the stairs. Next, I bumped her up the stairs to the living area of the house. She laughed all the way going up.

In addition to the living spaces upstairs, we had a screen-enclosed porch overlooking the backyard and pond. We would sit on the porch and listen to the wildlife while we visited. Mom especially enjoyed watching a couple of large horned owls that had taken up residence in our backyard. One day she got upset because they were fighting each other, and she wanted me to intervene. I explained, "We see them doing this each year. They are not fighting. It is their mating ritual."

We went to Biloxi one weekend and stayed at the Beau Rivage Resort & Casino. While we were there, we saw the Cirque de Soleil and dropped nickels into the slot machines.

Before I took her home, we went out one evening around Fairhope to look at the Christmas decorations. The colorful strands of multicolored lights signaled the approach of the celebration of the birth of Christ, which gives us hope and happiness. The lights also signaled Mom's return home. I was sad to see her leave, yet happy for her. It had been ten months since her stroke, and she was going where she wanted to be.

Looking back, I cannot think of a better time of the year for Mom to have fulfilled her desire. She had a fervent belief in God that she instilled in Michael and me. He got Mom home for Christmas, and He got me to state number fifty.

Once Mom was home, we hired two helpers. One came in the morning, prepared Mom's lunch, and placed it in the refrigerator. She also exercised Mom and cleaned the house. The second helper came in the evening, prepared Mom's dinner, and laid out the clothes Mom had selected to wear the next day. Mom did not spend the day sitting around in pajamas. She did not deviate from her prestroke daily routine. To do so would not have been normal.

She got up early, dressed herself, and fixed breakfast. She would stand at the sink washing breakfast dishes while looking out the window at the wildlife. A flock of turkeys came each day because of her handouts. She rode her battery-powered scooter around the yard, putting food in the bird feeders and in the gold-fish pond. Then she rode the scooter into the pasture among her cows. The scooter had thick wheels and would power through packed dirt but not deep sand.

Before I continue, let me introduce Sadie, an eighty-pound bulldog. Mom acquired the dog after its previous owner had mis-treated it. The dog adored Mom and was in a state of depres-sion during the ten months Mom was away. (A friend stayed at Mom's house and cared for Sadie.) Now, Sadie was excited over Mom's return.

One day, Mom was out in the pasture feeding pellets to her cows. Her scooter became stuck in loose soil. She had forgotten to charge her cell phone and could not call anyone. Fortunately, she had one of those life alert buttons. Soon the fire depart-ment, police department, and the newspaper showed up to help. However, Sadie would not allow them to get within ten feet of Mom. Eventually, they threw Mom a lasso that she looped over the back of the scooter, and they pulled her out. Sadie never left her side.

I continued my trips to visit each month. In the afternoons, Mom would take a nap and I would work in her yard or do other chores that she had on a list of things to do. In the late afternoon, we would get in the Jeep and drive around the ranch checking the cows. Sadie sat between us.

Things were good until Hurricane Frances came through Central Florida in September 2004. Michael, I, and our families were at the Jackson Lake Lodge in Wyoming. We were attend-ing the fourth International Conference on Relaxin and Related Peptides. Normally, Bushnell never had anything more than rain and light winds during a hurricane. However, this storm was a direct hit and knocked down power lines and trees. Roads were blocked, and Mom's helpers could not reach her. The first responders quickly worked to restore power and passage to Mom's house.

Mom took pleasure in monitoring the posthurricane restoration at Jumper Creek Ranch, and everything eventually returned to normal. Life was good again, at least for a while. Unfortunately, Hurricane Frances caused respiratory problems for people. This proved to be devastating to Mom. She came down with pneumonia and spent her last three months in a hospice in Gainesville.

On my second visit to the hospice, we talked about her returning home in time for Christmas. We even went down to the social room, where I played Christmas carols on the piano. My memory went back to the Christmas season in Fairhope, when we looked at Christmas lights prior to Mom going home. Like then, her spirits were high. On my next visit, her health had deteriorated, and it was obvious that she would not get back home a second time.

Typical of Mom, in her final days, she used a Christmas catalog and showed Michael what to buy family members for Christmas from her. In addition, she pointed out everyone working at the hospice for whom Michael was to buy a gift.

On December 8, 2004, Angels were picking flowers, and they took Mom.

Over Christmas, Michael and I took her gifts to the hospice and handed them out. There was not a dry eye in the hospice that day.

At the Catholic Church celebration of Mom's life, I presented the eulogy. As part of this, I borrowed and reworked a poem to express my feelings. Before I share that poem, I need to provide some background information.

The evening sky with the stars, Milky Way, and moon have always provided me with peace and hope. Several years before Mom's stroke, I presented her with a unique Mother's Day gift. I had purchased and named a star after Mom, Ann Ricica. Her parents had emigrated from Czechoslovakia. The family name, in Czechoslovakian, was Ricica. The star registry furnished a celestial map of the star's location. We often sat on her back patio at night and looked at it through a telescope.

Now, the poem.

A Star for Ann Ricica

So many hearts, so many lives,
You reached out and touched each one.
Your memories are all that's left for us,
We cherish each and every one.

I walk outside into the night,
And gaze up towards the sky.
There are no stars, the moon is gone,
I stand and wonder why.

Tears are flowing down my face,
My heart is aching so.
I search up high into the sky,
I ask, "Why did you have to go?"

Then through the darkness it appears,
One star that is so bright,
I swear it winked at me and said,
"Don't worry, I am all right."

With hope, I reach up to touch your face,
However, it's only the Milky Way.
I know you're where you want to be,
Yet I wish you could have stayed.

So every night that I go outside,
I know right where you are.
The brightest light God gave to you,
He called it, "Ann Ricica's Star."

Sadie died shortly after Mom. I believe she, too, was heartbroken.

We attempted to get the health department named after Mom, as a tribute to her love for Sumter County. The government works slowly, but sometimes it actually works. In 2013, nine years after Mom died, the State of Florida passed a resolution honoring the "Angel of Mercy." They also named County Road 476 in front of the Sumter County Health Clinic after Mom. A plaque with her photo adorns the wall in the clinic. Then, in 2019, the John Bartram Chapter of the Daughters of the American Revolution added Mom to its Women in Florida History.

Whenever I begin feeling sorry for myself and want to take the easier and more traveled road, I think about Mom. She had beaten the odds by challenging the limits that the stroke gave her. She told that neurologist "Bullshit" and spent five joyous years after the stroke in her own home, with her dog and her cows. These were her passions, her why, and they got her through.

Chapter Related Memory: Strawberry Short Cake.

One day, I told Mom that her smile reminded me of Uncle Lester.

One year (1967), my Aunt Mary, my Aunt Sylvia, and Aunt Sylvia's husband Lester drove down from their home in Ohio to Bushnell to visit us. We all then drove to Gainesville to visit Michael, who was in college at the University of Florida.

I had never known this group to drive past a Howard Johnson's restaurant without stopping for strawberry short-cake. So, on the way back to Bushnell, we stopped at a Howard Johnson's restaurant. Mom and Aunt Mary went inside to see if they had any strawberry shortcake. They would come get us if they had any. After a lengthy wait in the car, Aunt Sylvia, Lester, and I began to suspect foul play. Sure enough, the restaurant had only two slices of strawberry shortcake left. Mom and Aunt Mary were finishing them off as we walked into the restaurant to check on them. The two of them laughed and laughed over their trick-ery. I do not think Sylvia ever forgave them.

CHAPTER 33

The Raven

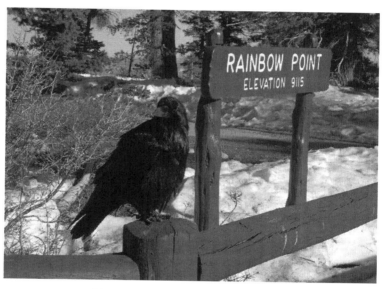

Bryce Canyon, Utah (2012)

Some say ravens point travelers in the right direction;
some say a single raven is a sight of good fortune to come.

Lucas E. Scott[34]

I have one final tribute—my favorite animal from my travels, the
raven. The raven is a majestic, soot-colored bird. It measures two
feet from the tip of its tail to the tip of its massive knifelike beak.

My first encounter with this bird was at the Tower of London (1988). The tour guide warned Mom, Leslie and me to keep our hands in our pockets, lest one of these birds remove a finger. The guide continued, "The raven developed a taste for human flesh ages ago when they feasted upon prisoners held at the Tower. These birds have passed the taste for this delicacy along to their offspring."

We were not sure if he was kidding about his last statement, although they do eat carrion. Nevertheless, we kept our hands securely in our pockets, and we each left the Tower with all ten of our fingers.

This bird was ever-present during our visits to state and national parks. I sensed it was my guardian angel, possibly sent by Mom. After all, I was with Mom the first time I encountered this bird in London. A strange echoing croak signals their presence. You will hear the sound long before you see the bird. It is opposite of seeing lightning before you hear the thunder.

At the Grand Canyon, I enjoyed glimpsing these winged beauties as they glided effortlessly across the sky above the Grand Canyon floor.

The raven is an extremely intelligent bird that will open backpacks or saddlebags on motorcycles in search of food. A treasure of any kind is appealing to this sneaky pickpocket. So be warned: Do not leave important items lying on a rock next to you. Otherwise, you will reach for your possession, only to find that the raven has claimed ownership.

A park ranger at Arches National Park told Marian and I about coming across a raven's treasure trove of plundered items. The bird's stash contained several thousand dollars' worth of trinkets: cameras, watches, jewelry, scarves, and even a set of car keys. The bird's treasure horde also contained prescription bottles with pills, billfolds, sunglasses, prescription glasses, and hats.

This inquisitive and confident bird will even take owner-ship of larger items that you would not normally worry about protecting from a bird, including vehicles (see photo below).

They are extremely comfortable in the presence of humans, and they strut (well, hop) around as if they are at the top of the food chain.

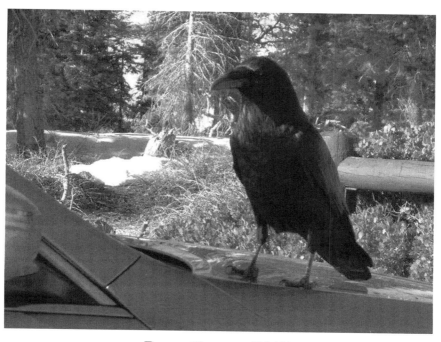

Bryce Canyon (2012)

While driving through Arches, I parked our rental car at the beginning of a hiking trail. Before beginning our hike, we took time to enjoy sandwiches we had purchased for lunch. I heard the croak. Then, out of nowhere, a large soot-colored raven dropped from the sky onto my side-view mirror. His intent was to share my sandwich. Actually, I believe he wanted it all. That crazy male bird was preparing to hop inside the car and onto the steering wheel. Thank goodness for electric windows.

That raven followed Marian and I to the next three stops along the park drive, ever vigilant for a handout.

(A word of caution: Do not feed animals in the wild since they will get used to handouts from humans and may fail to develop food stores for the winter.)

You are probably wondering how I knew that bird was a male. Short of doing a DNA test, it is difficult to tell the male from the female. Unlike most species of birds, the raven has no overt sexually dimorphic markings. On average, the male tends to be larger than the female. This was a huge bird, so I will refer to it as male.

If not for my intervention, an interesting event might have occurred at Bryce Canyon. I watched a man approach one of these massive birds as it was sitting on a post (see the chapter photo). The bird looked like a king watching over his realm. With camera in hand, the man eased closer to the bird for an up-close-and-personal photo. He was obviously unaware of what he was dealing with, so I called out, "I'm not sure I'd do that!"

I could have been silent, pulled out my cell phone, and filmed this YouTube-worthy moment. If we were concerned about our fingers at the Tower of London, there is no telling what this man might have lost.

We spoke briefly (the tourist and I, not the bird). He was under the impression that the bird was just a harmless crow. After our discussion, he backed away and used his zoom to capture the bird's photo. The bird remained on that post as calm as could be, as if he had been listening to our discussion while striking a pose for the tourist.

• • •

My high school English teacher (Mrs. Caruthers) had us read and discuss the meaning behind various books and poems. One of the poems was Edgar Allen Poe's "The Raven," first published in 1845. In high school, I was not the least bit interested in deciphering poems, especially one about a bird. However, with time, I have developed a fondness for this work. (I have bookmarked the poem on my computer and read it before each of my national park trips. The poem has made me appreciative of this black knight of our national parks.)

The poem tells of a talking raven's visit to a distraught lover and traces the man's slow descent into madness. The man sits reading forgotten lore, hoping to forget the loss of his love, Lenore. Suddenly, a talking raven enters his chambers. The man, who is also the narrator in the poem, moves close to admire this mysterious bird, sort of like the tourist at Bryce Canyon. While doing so, his mind wanders back to Lenore. He wonders if God is sending him a sign to forget her. The bird replies in the negative, "Nevermore," suggesting that the man can never be free of his memories.

To Poe, the raven was a symbol of mournful and never-ending remembrance. In Greek mythology, ravens are associated with Apollo, the god of prophecy. The Greeks believed them to be a symbol of good luck, acting as the god's messengers in the mortal world. I relate better to the Greek's symbolism of the raven since this bird has been an integral fixture in my journey.

As I reflect on my life, I see that it has been, symbolically, full of ravens. I feel like I have traveled in the right direction and have enjoyed many good fortunes. Thus, unlike the narrator in the poem, I do not want to be free of my memories, even if some of them are negative. In fact, there were numerous times during this journey when I asked myself, "Why do I continue? What good can ever come from this pain?" The answer to that question eluded me for years. Eventually, I looked beyond my own self-serving goals and my own self-pity in order to comprehend the solution: Take my suffering, and go help others.

There is a story about a man who fell down into a hole. As a physician walked by the hole, the man screamed, "Hey, doctor! I fell into this hole. Can you help me?" The doctor wrote out a prescription and threw it down into the hole.

Later a bishop walked by the hole. The man yelled, "Hey Monseigneur! I fell into this hole. Can you help me?" The bishop wrote out a prayer and threw it down into the hole.

Then, his friend walked by. The man cried out, "Hey, Joe! I fell into this hole. Can you help me?"

Joe jumped into the hole. The man said, "Nice going, Joe. Now there are two of us here," to which Joe replied, "Yes, but I've been in this hole before. I know the way out."

Alcoholics Anonymous learned a long time ago that the best way to help alcoholics who want to stop drinking is to put them in touch with someone who has been there. The Leukemia Lymphoma Society has a similar program, called First Connection, so I volunteered. Cancer is a hard battle to fight alone. Having a friend by your side through the countless appointments, the waiting for results, and the delivery of bad news is priceless. I have been there. I have done that.

Now, I can be a good listener. I can let people know they are not alone in their own personal battle. Maybe I can help provide hope when there is none or pick them up when they are down. Importantly, I can help them find their passion: things like reading, gardening, and watching sunrises, sunsets, the moon, and the stars.

It is especially important to find and exploit your passion during challenging times. After all, if you really want to live, you need to find something that makes life worth living. You need to find your "why."

In my journey, I have become keenly aware that the way you view a diagnosis—whether the prognosis is hopeful or less so—will greatly affect the time you have left to live. My diagnosis was definitely life changing. Yet I did not view it as an end but a beginning. I used my passion to my advantage and viewed leukemia as a blessing. Because of leukemia, I have gone places and seen sights I would not have experienced otherwise. Importantly, I learned more about myself, and I reached out to help others more than before.

There is a wonderful line by Ralph Waldo Emerson: "Do not go where the path my lead, go instead where there is no path and leave a trail."[35]

When I approach the end of my passage, I believe there are several criteria with which I can measure my journey's success. Did I create more carnage than good? Did I help someone through a difficult moment with a friendly comment? Did I open my heart to others, especially to God? Did I make the people I love smile and laugh? Lastly, do my good memories outweigh the bad ones?

Alternatively, has my journey been one of "Mournful and Never-ending Remembrances?" I have no doubt that my positive experiences far outweigh my sorrowful ones. God has blessed me with friends and family, and a passion that has helped me through difficult times.

For every single moment that has taken my breath away, I am truly grateful.

EPILOGUE

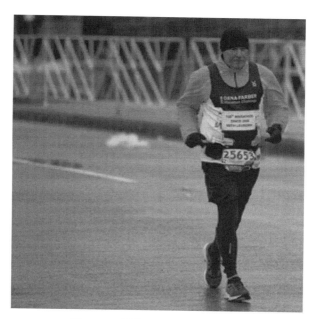

Boston Marathon (2018)

The ultimate measure of a man
is not where he stands in moments of comfort and convenience,
but where he stands at times of challenge and controversy.

Martin Luther King, Jr.[36]

A person goes through five stages upon hearing bad news and deal-ing with grief.[37]

    1. Denial: I certainly get a thumbs-up for this one. Upon hearing my diagnosis of leukemia, I spent six months

attempting to create a barrier that prevented my facing the reality that I had leukemia. I simply did not want to know what any of it meant.

2. Anger: "Why me?" "It's not fair." "What did I do to deserve this?"

I have never been one to blame others for what happens to me. I believe in taking ownership, and I skipped this phase.

3. Depression: I get a high five for this one. After the "knowing" shattered my wall of denial, I was body slammed by depression.

4. Bargaining: I certainly asked God for his help on numerous occasions during this journey. Yet, I did not promise that I would change my life if God helped rid me of leukemia. I never make a promise that I know I cannot keep.

5. Acceptance: Eventually, I accepted that I had leukemia and was not going to run marathons as I could before leukemia.

• • •

After four years driven by a goal to complete marathons in all fifty states and Washington, DC, my bucket was empty. I have seen so many people who retired and died shortly thereafter. I wondered, *Did they die because their bucket was empty? What if running marathons and sightseeing have helped me maintain my progression-free survival (time after treatment before the cancer returns). It at least has kept me from worrying about progression-free survival. This time bomb is still inside me, and I quickly need a new goal to silence the ticking.*

Even though I will not be able to qualify for the Boston Marathon again, I will not let leukemia rob me of my passion. After all, God went to a lot of trouble to make this beautiful planet. The least I can do is take the time and make the effort to enjoy his creation. Consequently, my next goals were to finish a marathon in the ten Canadian Provinces and the Civil War Battlefields.

Canadian Provinces

Manitoba Marathon (June 2013) in 5:30

Quebec City Marathon, Quebec (August 2013) in 5:38

Huffin' Puffin Marathon, Newfoundland (September 2013) in 5:31

Prince Edward Island (October 2013) in 5:00

Hamilton Marathon, Ontario (November 2013) in 5:27

Abbotsford, British Columbia (May 2014) in 5:10

Banff Marathon, Alberta (June 2014) in 6:10

Nova Scotia Marathon (July 2014) in 6:31

Saskatchewan Marathon (May 2015) in 5:26

Moncton, New Brunswick (October 2015) in 5:16

Civil War Battlefields

Chickamauga Marathon, GA (November 2014) in 6:02

Antietam, WV (October 2015) in 5:31

Gettysburg Marathon, PA (April 2016) in 5:57 (Book Spine Photo)

• • •

My real joy was returning to the Boston Marathon—twice. I entered both times through one of the Boston charities. The first time (April 2015, Book Cover Photo) was with the ALLY Foundation. Their mission is preventing sexual violence through science and innovation. I raised $10,000 and my finishing time was 5:19. The second time (April 2018) was with the Dana-Farber Cancer Institute. I raised $8,000 and my finishing time was 5:46. Both were spectacular moments that I will cherish.

I completed another goal at the 2018 Boston Marathon, my 100th marathon in 111 months since my leukemia diagnosis. I had hoped to accomplish this feat in as many months. However, I had to take three months off for removal of a melanoma and plastic surgery on my left calf (2014), five months off because of a heel fracture (2015), and another month off for a less extensive surgery to remove a melanoma from my right calf (2016).

I began having to completely stop running and walk the last eight to ten miles of a marathon. This issue was a result of the FCR chemotherapy. Because of damage to my heart, I was going into ventricular tachycardia at times and atrial fibrillation at other times.

In 2017, my cardiologist, and former student, Dr. John LeDoux, installed a defibrillator in my chest and encouraged me to find a new passion. He said, "You know you are going to drop dead in one of these marathons." After a year, John gave up on getting me to find a new passion. Now, he simply wishes me luck in being able to do what I love. I really like my cardiologist.

The smoothly paved marathon road that I started down in 1984 has become full of potholes. Now, I find it difficult running more than 0.2 of a mile in the last half of a marathon before having to stop and walk. A marathon is incredibly challenging when you hit the wall immediately after crossing the starting mat.

But, I have a new goal. Marian wants to run in all fifty states a second time, so I am simply going along for the ride in order to help her achieve her goal. After all, without her I would not have completed my goals or seen our beautiful country.

However, I am not obsessed with completing the states a second time. If I chose to drop out at the half during a marathon, I will not feel guilty. I will not carry any more monkeys.

Looking back, my journey from 1984 to the present has been so ironic. I never enjoyed the accomplishment of running marathons in the 3:30s because that time was not fast enough to qualify for the Boston Marathon. Then, after my diagnosis with leukemia, I failed to enjoy being able to run marathons in 4:30, then in 5:00, and eventually in 5:30. Now, I would love to be able to break 6:00 for a marathon.

Personally, I will never stop encouraging my students to establish where they want to be in life and never give up trying to get there. However, I have learned an important lesson: When a goal becomes an obsession, it can prevent you from thoroughly enjoying the journey.

Running continues to be my passion. Whatever setbacks I may encounter, I will savor whatever I now can accomplish running. As quoted by Ralph Waldo Emerson, "What lies behind you and what lies in front of you, pales in comparison to what lies inside of you."[38]

ABOUT THE AUTHOR

Phillip Arthur Fields received his BS degree from the University of Florida (1969) and his PhD in biochemistry from Texas A&M University (1976). He has been teaching human anatomy and human embryology to medical students at the University of South Alabama, College of Medicine in Mobile, Alabama since 1980. His desire is for his students to become successful doctors, and to have fun and enjoy the journey getting there. In 2007, an oncologist diagnosed him with leukemia, but he refused to let this blood cancer rob him of his passion-running marathons. He has completed over 100 marathons with leukemia, including one in every state and every Canadian Province. He has written this book with the hope that those diagnosed with cancer will never give up on living, and will find and hang on to their passion until the very end. He will donate all profits from this book to charitable organizations including pediatric oncology.

PERSONAL ACKNOWLEDGEMENTS

Chelsea Adams, Starlight Editorial, Mobile, Alabama, for her excellent editing of this document. Each time I thought I was finished, she challenged me to add, delete, or clarify details in my personal stories. Her website is Chelsea@starlighteditorial. com. She provides proofreading of transcripts for court reporters; checking grammar and spelling, and deep analysis of characters and plot for authors; editing brochures, newsletters, essays, memos and websites to be sure they are polished and on brand for professionals.

Jon Fredrick, Boston Massachusetts, for the front-cover-page photo. He took the photo while I was in Boston for the 2015 Boston Marathon. Jon offers professional services for weddings, engagements, commercial, events/sporting and landscapes. His website: http://jonfrederickphotography.zenfolio.com/

Dr. Thomas Butler, my hematologist-oncologist (Mitchell Cancer Institute, Mobile, AL). I love Dr. Butler's holistic and conservative approach to dealing with my leukemia. He is always optimistic and reassuring about outcome. I consider him a friend.

Dr. John LeDoux, my cardiologist (Cardiology Associates, Mobile, AL). He worries about me running marathons with my heart condition. Even though I will not listen to his advice to quit running them, he continues to do everything in his power to help me sustain my passion. I consider him a friend as well.

END NOTES

1   James Dean Quotes. BrainyQuote.com, Xplore Inc, 2018.
https://www.brainyquote.com/quotes/james_dean_103528.

2   https://www.azquotes.com/author/10976-Frank_O_Hara.

3   H. P. Lovecraft Quotes. BrainyQuote.com, Xplore Inc, 2018.
https://www.brainyquote.com/quotes/h_p_lovecraft_676245.

4   Colin Powell Quotes. BrainyQuote.com, Xplore Inc, 2018.
https://www.brainyquote.com/quotes/colin_powell_137376.

5   Praagh, V. https://www.pinterest.com/VanPraagh/
inspirational-quotes/?lp=true.

6   Nadine Daher. QuotesWave.com.
http://www.quoteswave.com/textquotes/413966.

7   Elodie Yung Quotes. BrainyQuote.com, Xplore Inc, 2018.
https://www.brainyquote.com/quotes/elodie_yung_756428.

8   Leo Buscaglia Quotes. BrainyQuote.com, Xplore Inc, 2018.
https://www.brainyquote.com/quotes/leo_buscaglia_143453.

9   Blake, W. http://quoteseverlasting.com/author.
php?a=William%20Blake

10   Lincoln, A. https://www.thoughtco.com/
abraham-lincoln-quotations-everyone-should-know-1773576.

11   Napoleon Hill Quotes. BrainyQuote.com, Xplore Inc, 2018.
https://www.brainyquote.com/quotes/napoleon_hill_152843.

12   Albert Camus Quotes. BrainyQuote.com, Xplore Inc, 2018. https://www.brainyquote.com/quotes/albert_camus_100779.

13   Harburg, EY. https://www.goodreads.com/author/quotes/5758090.E_Y_Harburg.

14   Pam Brown Quotes. Jar of Quotes, 2018. https://www.jarofquotes.com/view.php?id=dreams-are-journeys-that-take-one-far-from-familiar-shores-strengthening-the-heart-empowering-the-soul.

15   Bombeck, E. https://www.goodreads.com/quotes/8499-seize-the-moment-remember-all-those-women-on-the-titanic.

16   Elko, K. https://www.tuscaloosanews.com/opinion/20110501/dr-kevin-elko-finding-the-highest-questions-after-a-disaster.

17   Parkes, CM (1998). Bereavement in Adult Life. BMJ 316 (7134) 856-859.

18   Robin S. Sharma Quotes. BrainyQuote.com, Xplore Inc, 2018. https://www.brainyquote.com/quotes/robin_s_sharma_628740.

19   Saint Augustine Quotes. BrainyQuote.com, Xplore Inc, 2018. https://www.brainyquote.com/quotes/saint_augustine_108132.

20   Marcus Aurelius Quotes. BrainyQuote.com, Xplore Inc, 2018. https://www.brainyquote.com/quotes/marcus_aurelius_143090.

21   Lewis, CS. https://www.deseretnews.com/top/817/0/Top-100-CS-Lewis-quotes-.html.

22   Cabot, M. https://www.azquotes.com/quote/345224.

23   Michelangelo Quotes. BrainyQuote.com, Xplore Inc, 2018. https://www.brainyquote.com/quotes/michelangelo_108779.

24   Brian Tracy Quotes. BrainyQuote.com, BrainyMedia Inc, 2018. https://www.brainyquote.com/quotes/brian_tracy_125679.

25   Corona, V. https://quoteinvestigator.com/2013/12/17/breaths/.

26   Einstein, A. https://www.goodreads.com/quotes/987-there-are-only-two-ways-to-live-your-life-one

27   Mother Teresa. https://www.goodreads.com/quotes/477617-we-learn-humility-through-accepting-humilia-tions-cheerfully.

28   Praagh, JV. https://www.goodreads.com/author/quotes/40330.

29   Ralph Waldo Emerson Quotes. BrainyQuote.com, Xplore Inc, 2018.
https://www.brainyquote.com/quotes/ralph_waldo_emerson_385779.

30   Praagh, JV.https://www.goodreads.com/quotes/225675-i-drather-look-forward-and-dream-than-look-backward-and

31   McFarland, JH. http://www.presidency.ucsb.edu/ws/index.php?pid=19920.

32   Napoleon Hill Quotes. BrainyQuote.com, Xplore Inc, 2018.
https://www.brainyquote.com/quotes/napoleon_hill_121370.

33   Suenens, LJ. https://www.goodreads.com/quotes/24905-hope-is-not-a-dream-but-a-way-of-making.

34   Scott, L. http://www.searchquotes.com/quotation/Some_say_ravens_point_travelers_in_the_right_direction%2C_some_say_a_single_raven_is_a_sight_of_good_f/248982/.

35   Ralph Waldo Emerson Quotes. BrainyQuote.com, Xplore Inc, 2018.
https://www.brainyquote.com/quotes/ralph_waldo_emerson_101322.

36   Martin Luther King, Jr. Quotes. BrainyQuote.com, Xplore Inc, 2018.
https://www.brainyquote.com/quotes/martin_luther_king_jr_109228.

37   Williams-Murphy M, Murphy K. (2011) It's Okay to Die. The Authors and MKN, LLC.

38   Ralph Waldo Emerson Quotes. BrainyQuote.com, BrainyMedia Inc, 2018.
https://www.brainyquote.com/quotes/ralph_waldo_emerson_386697.